Counseling & Diversity

Counseling Latino/a Americans

Michele R. Guzmán
The University of Texas at Austin

Nicolás Carrasco
Clinical and Forensic Psychology
Austin, TX

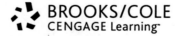
BROOKS/COLE
CENGAGE Learning™

Australia • Brazil • Japan • Korea • Mexico • Singapore • Spain • United Kingdom • United States

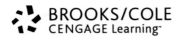
BROOKS/COLE
CENGAGE Learning™

Counseling & Diversity,
Counseling Latino/a Americans
Michele R. Guzmán and Nicolás Carrasco

Series Editors: Devika Dibya Choudhuri and
  Azara Santiago-Rivera

Acquisitions Editor: Seth Dobrin

Associate Development Editor: Nic Albert

Assistant Editor: Naomi Dreyer

Editorial Assistant: Suzanna Kincaid

Marketing Manager: Christine Sosa

Marketing Communications Manager:
  Tami Strang

Production Manager: Matt Ballantyne

Art Director: Caryl Gorska

Print Buyer: Judy Inouye

Rights Acquisition Specialist, Text:
  Bob Kauser

Rights Acquisition Specialist, Art:
  Don Schlotman

Production Service: PreMedia Global

Compositor: PreMedia Global

For product information and technology assistance, contact us at
Cengage Learning Customer & Sales Support, 1-800-354-9706

For permission to use material from this text or product,
submit all requests online at **www.cengage.com/permissions**
Further permissions questions can be emailed to
permissionrequest@cengage.com

Library of Congress Control Number: 2011921177

ISBN-13: 978-0-618-47044-0

ISBN-10: 0-618-47044-1

Brooks/Cole
20 Davis Drive
Belmont, CA 94002
USA

Cengage Learning is a leading provider of customized learning solutions with
office locations around the globe, including Singapore, the United Kingdom,
Australia, Mexico, Brazil, and Japan. Locate your local office at
www.cengage.com/global

Cengage Learning products are represented in Canada by
Nelson Education, Ltd.

To learn more about Brooks/Cole, visit **www.cengage.com/brookscole**

Purchase any of our products at your local college store or at our preferred
online store **www.cengagebrain.com**

Printed in the United States of America
2 3 4 5 6   19 18 17 16 15

To Guadalupe Saldivar Guzmán, for her courage,
her love, and the doors that she opened for me.
And To Bernardino and Natalia Saldivar, for connecting me
with my culture. Your spirits live on in this book.

CONTENTS

5 Counseling Dynamics and Interventions   79

6 Resource List for Further Reading   101

PREFACE

This book is the work of two psychologists, a *Latina* and a *Latino*. Throughout this book, we will share with you our histories, our families, and our lives—our *Latinidad* ("Latino-ness")—in order to concretize for you the Latino experience in the United States. Through this sharing, we hope to help you know—in the true sense of the word—Latino culture.

In this monograph, you will learn that our roots in this country run deep, and that our Indigenous ancestors established themselves in this hemisphere thousands of years ago. They evolved into great civilizations centuries ago, only to be destroyed by our European ancestors and then rebuilt by the blood, sweat, and tears of our African ancestors. We are, therefore, of all shades and colors: black, white, brown, red, light, dark, and in-between. We are *negritos, prietos, morenos, trigueños, gueros.* We are Latinos; we are *La Raza,* the Cosmic Race (Vasconcelos, 1979).

We will present our history and how we have treated each other. Latinos are at once the conquerors and the conquered, the masters and the slaves, the rich and the poor, the privileged and the underprivileged. We have hurt each other and have done so with great cruelty, and we have helped each other heal and have done so with great compassion. Ours has been, and still is, a great struggle, and in that struggle we sacrifice much and do so willingly. We work, and we do so inexhaustibly. We share, and we do so generously. We have great respect for our elders, a strong sense of obligation to our family, and a deep, deep faith in our deities. You will learn what unites us and what divides us. You will become familiar with our worldviews and our cultural realities. You will begin to know the essence of being Latino.

OUR JOURNEYS

Nicolás...

My journey into ethnicity began in San Juan, in the Rio Grande Valley of Texas. On the southwest corner of 2nd and Kansas is a lot where stood a two-bedroom house in the front, and three one-room shacks in the back. The middle shack had a tin roof and the interior got blistering hot under the south Texas summer sun. I was born in that shack on August 23, 1954, oblivious to all that I was and ignorant of all that I was to become.

In San Juan, I was raised and lived as a *Mexicano*. There I lived the traditional Mexicano life, and I learned our *costumbres* (customs) and our values. In San Juan, I heard and celebrated mass in Latin, in one of the most venerated Catholic churches in the country. On bended knee I witnessed the actions of deep faith; not my own, but that of my people who made their way on their knees from the street, up the steps of the cathedral, and down the long aisle to the altar where they fulfilled their *promesas* (promises) to God in return for a miracle. I lived across the street from the beloved and respected *curandera* (healer), Doña Tomasita, and I was healed by her several times of ailments such as *mal de ojo* ("evil eye"; see p. 108) and *susto* (fright). In San Juan, I watched my father become deathly ill; when no doctors could diagnose and treat his ailment, a *curandero* from Reynosa removed the *embrujo* (evil spell), and my father still lived during the writing of this book.

In San Juan, I learned the importance of extended family and *compadres* (coparents), and respect for my elders. In San Juan, I learned Spanish before I learned English, and I learned about Antonio Aguilar, Javier Solis, and Jose Alfredo Jimenez before I learned about Roy Rogers, Gene Autry, and Tex Ritter. I learned about *El Rayo de Plata* (Silver Lightning) before I learned about Superman or Batman, and I learned about *Chucho el Roto* before I learned about Robin Hood. In San Juan, I learned to be *macho* before I was a man.

We were migrant farm workers, and I learned to work before I learned to play. I learned to pick cotton before I learned to identify colors. In the potato and cucumber fields of west Texas I learned to count sacks before I learned to multiply and divide in school. In the migrant labor camps, I learned to work hard and to value education. I saw discrimination.

In the government housing projects of Harlingen and Edinburg, Texas, I learned that we were poor, and in poverty I learned about friendship, about sharing, and about interdependence. I learned about sacrifice and about pride, and became a Mexican American.

In Austin, Texas, I learned that I was a minority, and learned about prejudice, my own and others'. I learned about myself and my people, and I was able to put my prejudice aside and replace it with righteous anger, and ultimately with legitimate power. I became a *Chicano*, and in doing so, I learned to fight for the cause by helping Chicano and minority youth.

In the 1980s, after years of living as a Chicano, I noticed a new term begin to emerge—"Hispanic." In fact, the 1980s were designated as "The Decade of the Hispanics," and demographers and statisticians began to predict that Hispanics would soon be the largest minority group in the United States. Use of the term "Hispanic" became commonplace, and I was referred to as "Hispanic." This label, however, felt imposed on me by the government and the media. It did not "fit" me exactly, and I did not embrace it. I sensed, however, from the manner in which it was used that the community at large—the United States—was beginning to take notice and to recognize the presence and importance of our people, and I liked that. "*Ya era tiempo;* it's about time," I thought.

As predicted, the Hispanic population did continue to grow, and over the last twenty years and into the new millennium, Hispanics in the United States have become a driving force—a dynamic, energetic movement of people with cultural roots in Mexico, Central America, South America, and the Caribbean. I count myself an active and vibrant part of that movement. Together we Hispanics are finding our voice, and we chose a name for ourselves: not Hispanic, not Latin, but Latino. I am Latino. I am comfortable with this designation, not because it fits me as neatly as Chicano but because it comes from our people. I am third generation Latino; I am Chicano; I am Mexican American; I am Mexicano. I invite you to know me as I know myself.

Michele...

My experience of being Mexican American has been one of being highly acculturated, but maintaining a strong ethnic identity. I was born in Austin, Texas. My great-grandparents were born in Mexico. Both sets of grandparents were born in Texas, but grew up speaking Spanish. My parents were the first generation to receive a formal education. They recall being hit on the hands with rulers for speaking Spanish in school. They were able to move away from the Rio Grande Valley and attend the University of Texas at Austin.

My parents bought the American Dream lock, stock, and barrel. They built a house in a predominately White European American neighborhood and only spoke English to us at home. Until their divorce, which brought with it more difficult economic times, I remember being able to order every book in the Scholastic book catalog. The importance of education was instilled in us from the beginning.

My maternal grandparents were our daycare, after-school care, and summer camp. They spoke only Spanish, but due to their lack of education they passed on to us a sometimes amusing "Espanglish." Along with the language came traditions, food, and stories about their upbringing, and visits to the Valley to see relatives on both sides of the family; these were my ties to the culture. I felt comfortable eating tacos and tamales, but remember thinking that the interiors of our relatives' houses in the Valley, with their altars and plastic coverings on the furniture, didn't look like our house. I thought it was funny that I identified as Mexican American, but when I would ask my grandmother—who couldn't even carry on a conversation in English—how she identified, she would say "American." I didn't understand then the discrimination that would lead her to want to distance herself from her Mexican roots. I also learned that she was "American" in so many ways. As I began to learn Spanish more formally in school, I would sometimes look to my grandmother for help. Once, when I wanted to know the Spanish word for "tape," she racked her brain and then replied, "*Pues, escotch tape.*" The same thing happened when I inquired about the Spanish word for "bleach": she answered with "*Clorox*"—but with an accent, mind you.

I went through elementary school thinking that we, along with two other friends in my neighborhood, were the only Hispanics around. That all changed with desegregation, when I was bussed to East Austin and realized that there were a lot of us. But at the same time, I was different. The Mexican-origin students from East Austin resented my advantages and let me know that I wasn't as Mexican as they were. From this experience came a lifetime of trying to figure out where I fit in. I knew I wasn't White, but I wasn't Mexican either. I've spent many years improving my Spanish, making trips to Mexico, and reconnecting with my Mexican American heritage. Through my graduate work in multicultural counseling, my research about ethnic identity and educational struggles among Mexican Americans, and my work in diversity education, I have come to define for myself what being Mexican American means to me. My experiences have shaped me, but I've come to recognize that there is no single legitimate experience of being Mexican American. My experience is unique, as is the experience of each Latino or Latina.

ACKNOWLEDGMENTS

A special acknowledgment to Azara Santiago-Rivera, Melba Vásquez and Manuel Ramírez III for their support and mentorship; also to Rick Ybarra for his ongoing encouragement and helpful feedback on the revisions.

We are indebted to our families who were supportive during the book's preparation and revision. Our sincere gratitude to Irma and Cristal Carrasco, Pedro Guzmán, Jr., Jose Luis Garcia, Monica Guzmán, and Melissa Guzmán for their unwavering support and assistance, and to Millicent Villela and Paul-Michael Guzmán for their love. A special thanks to David Greiner and Peter R. Guzmán who provided the love, caring, and faith that saw this book to its completion and to Nicolas and Noemi Greiner-Guzmán for their patience and love when the revision of this book took time and attention away from them.

CHAPTER 1

Demographic Profile of Latinos in the United States

INTRODUCTION

Latinos are a diverse group of people, not only in terms of national origin, but with respect to many other characteristics. They differ dramatically in areas such as educational attainment, socioeconomic status, age, religion, and employment. Latinos have ancestral roots in over thirty different countries. It is especially important to pay close attention to these demographic variables as they relate to your client. Variables such as the highest level of education achieved and annual income will influence how an individual experiences his or her ethnic culture. We begin by addressing labels with which Latinos may identify.

TERMINOLOGY

One of the first concerns that counselors-in-training often express is a fear of offending clients simply through the terminology used to address them. While ethnic self-labeling, as well as self-identification concerning other identities, is a personal preference, it is good to have an understanding of the issues surrounding terminology for any given group with whom you might work. There has been considerable debate in the literature about whether "Latino" or "Hispanic" is the most appropriate term for this pan-ethnic group. For reasons that will be made clear below, neither term is entirely accurate (Gonzalez, 2000). Despite this shortcoming, we consider them to be the most inclusive terms, and for convenience rather than accuracy we will use them interchangeably in this text. In the following sections, we hope to familiarize you with the issues behind this debate and give you some guidance in how to address concerns over self-labeling in this group.

Hispanics, Latinos, or Neither?

Students and service providers unfamiliar with Latinos often struggle with the variety of terms used to refer to people in the United States who are themselves, or whose ancestors were, from a Spanish-speaking country. There is confusion and sometimes apprehension that a person may use a term that a client may find offensive. The group as a whole is often referred to as "Latino" or "Hispanic," while various subgroup names are also used (e.g. Mexican, Mexican American, Puerto Rican, etc.). Group names with political significance are also used (e.g. La Raza, Chicanos, "*Boriquas*," etc.). Mistakenly, people often think that the choice of term is simply a matter of present-day political correctness. In reality, a preference for a particular term involves historical significance, political consciousness, and personal preference.

It is important to note that the terms "Latino" and "Hispanic" are pan-ethnic labels, referring collectively to people from a variety of ethnic backgrounds. These terms do not refer to racial groups. Latino and Hispanic are not races as we commonly conceive racial groups in the United States. In reality, Latinos or Hispanics are of mixed racial heritage, made up of Black, White, and Indigenous roots. Terms such as "Mexican American," "Dominican," or "Cuban American" are ethnic terms and refer to groups of people from a particular country or with ancestors from a specific country.

Hispanic

"Hispanic" is another term for "Spanish," which literally refers to people from Spain. The current use of the term in the United States is somewhat analogous to the use of the word "Anglo," which literally refers to people from England. The word "Anglo" has been applied to groups which are now more often referred to as "White" or "European American," but it should be noted that "White" is a racial term, while "European American" is a pan-ethnic label. Similarly, in the United States we have come to use the term "Hispanic" to refer to anyone and anything that is remotely related to anything Spanish. For example, the term can be applied equally to label a first-generation Spanish-speaking Afro-Cuban living in New York or a White English-speaking sixth-generation Californian of Mexican descent. The term "Hispanic" received official government sanction in 1968 when President Johnson declared the week of September 15 to be "National Hispanic Week," at the prompting of Senator Joseph Montoya of New Mexico (Melville, 1994). Historically, the term "Hispanic" (as opposed to "Mexican" or "Mexican American") has always had greater use and acceptance in New Mexico. There is a community of people there who hold strongly to their Spanish roots, some of which date back to 1598. After 1968, the term "Hispanic" came into greater use.

In 1980 the federal Office of Management and Budget began to use the term "Hispanic" on United States Census forms. On census surveys conducted between 1950 and 1970, Hispanics had been identified as "White person of Spanish surname," "White," and "Spanish/Hispanic"

(Hayes-Bautista and Chapa, 1987). These labels grouped this diverse group into one racial category and ignored their specific countries of origin. The 1970 census was the first to recognize nationality (e.g. Puerto Rican) among Hispanics, but also confused the issue by mixing in Spanish surname and language as equivalent identifiers. On the 1980 and 1990 census forms, "Spanish/Hispanic" origin people had the opportunity to identify more closely with their country of origin or with other forms of ethnic self-identification (such as Chicano or Mexican American). With respect to race, since 1970, Latinos have been the only group to have a racial group membership question separate from the one about ethnicity, but like everyone else, could only select one racial group. Beginning in 2000 and again in 2010, Latinos could select "one or more races," not only reflecting their diversity, but also creating some confusion after so many years of only being able to select one group. The 2000 census form was the first to include the term "Latino," in the question "Is Person … Spanish/Hispanic/Latino," again followed by an opportunity to further self-identify with respect to ethnic group (U.S. Department of Commerce, Bureau of the Census, 2000). In 2010 the wording changed slightly to "Is Person … of Hispanic, Latino, or Spanish origin" (U.S. Department of Commerce, Bureau of the Census, 2010).

The U.S. government is not alone in struggling to find an appropriate label for this diverse group. Latinos themselves have conflicting feelings regarding which term is preferable. "Hispanic" is a term that some people dislike because it connotes a cultural heritage related to Spain, and the term is thus thought to reflect a history of colonization, assimilation, and exploitation of Indigenous peoples by a "superior" European power (Granados, 2000; Falicov, 1998). In addition, some people find the term objectionable because it was chosen for—or imposed on—the group by the U.S. government, and as a result the term may be experienced as further colonization. Furthermore, the use of "Hispanic" presumes not only a common language (Spanish) but also a common national heritage (Spain). In this regard, it fails to recognize the immense diversity of the population that immigrated (voluntarily or otherwise) and contributed significantly to the development of the New World, a group that included millions of people from Africa, Italy, France, Portugal, Germany, Ireland, and elsewhere (Santiago-Rivera, Arredondo, and Gallardo-Cooper, 2002).

Latino

Some people prefer to use the term "Latino," which is derived from the word "Latin," the language of the Roman Empire. Modern-day Spain was part of the Roman Empire, and Spanish is derived from ancient Latin. Thus, the term "Latino" is better suited, than the term "Hispanic", to describe the national origins or ancestry of the vast majority of the people who reside in "Latin America": Mexico, Central and South America, and the Spanish-speaking regions of the Caribbean. "Latino" is also derived from *latinoamerica*, the Spanish word for Latin America; it is more of a self-imposed (rather than government-imposed) ethnic label, making it is easier for people to accept (Gonzalez, 1992) despite its association with Europe, the conquest, and all the negative repercussions of that chapter in our history. Some authors suggest that "Latino" better differentiates people of Latin American and Caribbean descent (Spanish mixed with African and Indigenous influences) from those who come to the U.S. from Spain or are only of Spanish origin (Hayes-Bautista & Chapa, 1987).

However, it should be noted that regardless of the points presented earlier, many people from this group still prefer the term "Hispanic." Because the term has been around longer than "Latino," it is for many the more familiar or comfortable term, the one that people see more often on demographic forms, and the term often passed down from one generation to another without any particular rationale. A national survey ($N = 2929$) conducted jointly by the Pew Hispanic Center and the Kaiser Family Foundation (2002) found that a majority of the Latino participants (53%) indicated that they do not have a preference between the terms "Latino" and "Hispanic," but of the 47% who did, Hispanic (34%) was generally preferred to "Latino" (14%).

Pan-Ethnic Versus Ethnic-Specific Labels

One of the advantages of the terms "Hispanic" and "Latino" is that they are useful for referring collectively to people from a variety of ethnic backgrounds, but this is also one of their major shortcomings. Both "Latino" and "Hispanic" are pan-ethnic labels. "Panethnicity" refers "to the development of solidarity among ethnic groups" (Schaefer, 2002, p. 272): a shared sense of identity or Latinidad (De Genova & Ramos-Zayas, 2003). There is some indication that panethnicity is developing prominence in the Spanish-language media (television and periodicals). By and large, however, sharp divisions remain, and research suggests that only one in four Latinos "prefer to use pan-ethnic names such as *Hispanic* or *Latino* or *Spanish American....* [T]he majority prefer identifying themselves by nationality—*Mexican, Mexican American, Chicanos, Puerto Ricans, Cubans and Dominicans*" (Schaefer, 2002, p. 274). Results of the national survey mentioned previously (Pew Hispanic Center and the Kaiser Family Foundation; 2002) also indicate that a little more than half of the participants (54%) preferred to first identify themselves with a term specifying country of origin or ancestry (e.g. Cuban, Dominican, Mexican, Colombian, etc.). Only 24% chose "Latino" or "Hispanic" as a primary label, and 21% percent self-identified first as simply "American." The Pew study did not appear to investigate preferences for identification with terms that politically affirm one's ethnic identity, such as "Chicano" or "Boricua," which may also be the preference of some Latinos (Comas-Díaz, 2001).

Summary

The terms "Hispanic" and "Latino" both have positives and negatives, and research suggests that at this time Hispanics or Latinos do not strongly prefer one to the other. The term "Latino" is preferred by the authors of this text, although for the reasons stated earlier in the chapter we use the term with some reservation. Furthermore, it may be best to use specific ethnic designations when speaking with individuals, reserving the use of pan-ethnic labels for situations that make reference to the Latino population as a whole or to several communities at once.

Students often wonder, with all these information in mind, how one is supposed to know which term a client prefers. The answer is simple: ask the client. A question such as "How do you identify ethnically?" or some variation will usually suffice. Asking a client such a question also allows a counselor to collect information on whether or not ethnic identification is even important to the client, a topic which will be discussed further in Chapter 4.

LATINO POPULATION

This book is going into production as the 2010 census data are being entered and analyzed, but the 2008 American Community Survey provided a statistical portrait of the 304 million residents living in the U.S. at that time, 46.8 million (or 15.4%) were Hispanic. Of these, 60% were "native born" (born in the U.S.) and 40% were foreign born (Pew Hispanic Center, 2010). This number is up from the 35.2 million Hispanics reported from 2000 census data, 12.5% of the total U.S. population at the time. People of Hispanic origin are the largest ethnic or racial minority in the U.S. There was a 3.1% increase in the Hispanic population between July 1, 2008 and July 1, 2009, making Hispanics the fastest-growing minority group (U.S. Census Bureau, 2010a). In 2000 the Census Bureau predicted that by the year 2050 the number of Latinos in the U.S. would constitute a full 25% of the population (Schaefer, 2002). That prediction has now been revised to 30%, or a projected 132.8 million (U.S. Census Bureau, 2010a).

"Latin America" is comprised of over thirty countries, counting the numerous island nations found in the Caribbean, and the Latino population in the U.S. can trace their ancestry to one or more of these countries. As will be discussed in the next chapter, Latinos of Mexican, Cuban, and Puerto Rican descent have had a long and significant presence in this country. More recently, "other Latino" groups—from South America, Central America, and the Dominican Republic—have figured prominently in U.S. culture (Guzmán, 2001).

Of the 46.8 million Latinos counted in the American Community survey in 2008, those of Mexican origin represented 66%, of Puerto Rican ancestry 9%, and of Cuban background 3.4%. Latinos of Salvadoran background made up another 3.4%, and those of Dominican descent 2.8%. The remainder were of other Central American, South American, Hispanic, or Latino origin (U.S. Census Bureau, 2010a). While people of Mexican origin are the largest group of Latinos in the U.S., other Latino groups have experienced large growth rates during the last two decades. A study conducted by the Pew Hispanic Center (2002) indicates that between 1990 and 2000 there was a 140.6% increase in the Honduran population in the U.S. Large increases were also observed in the Guatemalan (99.0%), Dominican (80.4%), and Ecuadorian

(81.6%) populations. Other Latino subgroups also had large increases, though not as dramatic.

AGE

The 2008 American Community Survey results indicate that the median age for the entire U.S. population was 36.8 years, but that for Latinos it was just 27.4 years (Pew Hispanic Center, 2010). Data from the 2000 census showed that 35% of Latinos were under age 18, while only 25.7% of the U.S. population as a whole fell below this age. By 2008, Latinos comprised 22% of all children under age 18. It is significant that this population is so young: Latinos are our future. They are the voters, taxpayers, consumers, and potentially the leaders of the next generation. It would benefit the nation to think carefully about how to best invest in these young people. It should be noted that Cubans differ significantly from the other Latino groups with respect to age. They have a median age of 40.1, and also have a much greater percentage (17.7%) of people over 65 years old than other Latino groups, where this figure ranges from 4.4% (Mexican Americans) to 7.6% for "Other Hispanic" (Guzmán, 2001).

GEOGRAPHIC LOCATION

Nearly half of all Latinos in the U.S. live in just two states: California and Texas. The seven states with the largest Latino populations are California, Texas, New York, Florida, Illinois, Arizona, and New Jersey, with 74% of Latinos living in these areas (Pew Hispanic Center, 2010). Data show that Latinos of specific ethnic origins tend to cluster in certain areas of the country. The largest populations of people of Mexican descent are concentrated in California, Texas, Illinois, and Arizona. The largest concentrations of Puerto Rican individuals are in New York, Florida, New Jersey, and Pennsylvania. About two-thirds of all people of Cuban descent live in Florida. Dominicans tend to concentrate in the northeast, where 85% live (Guzmán, 2001). Central and South Americans tend to settle in cities where there are large numbers of other Latinos, like Miami, Los Angeles, New York, San Francisco, and Washington, D.C. (Hernandez, 2004). Some of the traditional Latino destination sites (Dallas, Riverside-San Bernadino) saw growth rates of over 300% in the last twenty years. Houston, Orange County, and Phoenix all saw growth over 200%. A relatively new phenomenon is the "hypergrowth" experienced by many "New Latino Destinations" in the last twenty years. For example, Raleigh, North Carolina recorded a growth rate of 1180% in its Latino population. Atlanta, Greensboro, and Charlotte experienced growth rates over 900%; and an additional fourteen sites across the U.S. saw Latino populations increase by between 300% and 800%. Latinos are no longer concentrated only in the traditional areas of the Southwest, New York, and Florida: they are establishing communities in all parts of the country (Center on Urban and Migration Policy; The Pew Hispanic Center, 2002).

EMPLOYMENT AND WAGES

In March 2002, only 5% of non-Latino Whites aged 16 and older in the civilian labor force were unemployed, compared with 8.1% of Latinos (U.S. Census Bureau, 2002). With the economic downturn that began in late 2008, unemployment among all groups rose sharply. July 2010 data show the non-Hispanic White civilian labor force experiencing an unemployment rate of 8.7%, while Latinos were at 12.2% and African Americans at 16.6% (U.S. Department of Labor, 2010). Latinos are also more likely than non-Latino Whites to work in service occupations: 22.1% and 11.6%, respectively. Only 14.2% of Latinos were in professional or managerial occupations, compared with 35.1% of non-Latino Whites (U.S. Census Bureau, 2002).

Given the lack of adequate employment, it follows that there is also a marked discrepancy in household income when comparing Latinos to non-Latino Whites. In 2008, the median income for all races was $51,938. For Whites, that number was $56,826, but for Hispanics the median household income was $41,041 (Pew Hispanic Center, 2010). The National Survey of Latinos ($N = 2929$; Pew Hispanic Center & Kaiser Family Foundation, 2002) found that native-born Latinos (those born in the U.S.) tended to have higher household incomes than foreign-born Latinos, and data from 2008 demonstrate that this trend continues with foreign-born Latinos having a medium income of $38,699 compared with that of $45,828 for native-born Latinos (Pew Hispanic Center). The same discrepancy was observed for Latinos who primarily speak English, or are bilingual, compared to those who primarily speak Spanish, with the first group reporting higher incomes than the second.

POVERTY AND WEALTH

In 2008, 23.2% of Latinos were living in poverty, compared to 8.2% of non-Latino Whites (U.S. Census Bureau, 2010a). The discrepancy in child poverty is even more severe, with 26.4% of Latino children younger than age 18 living in poverty, compared with only 10% of non-Latino White children (Pew Hispanic Center, 2010). As has been the case with other demographic variables, poverty rates for different Latino groups vary widely. Puerto Ricans have the greatest number of families living below the poverty line (26.1%), while 22.8% of families of Mexican descent and 16.5% of Cuban families live in poverty. There are slightly fewer South and Central American families (15.2%) living below the poverty level; however, this is still higher than the overall poverty rate for non-Latino Whites (Ramirez & de la Cruz, 2002).

A report released by the Pew Hispanic Center indicated that the difference in wealth between Latinos and non-Latino Whites was even greater than the difference in household income. The report states, "Hispanic households have less than ten cents for every dollar in wealth owned by White households.... But even the wealthiest five percent of Hispanic households have a net worth that is less than one-half of the net worth of comparably placed White households" (Kochhar, 2004, p. 1). In essence, Latinos live from paycheck to paycheck. As might be expected, poverty influences many other areas of present-day life, such as housing, diet, educational opportunity, and health care, while the lack of wealth denies Latinos the ability to "get ahead" by means such as starting their own businesses. They also lack less tangible opportunities, such as travel or academic and cultural enrichment experiences for their children.

RISE OF THE MIDDLE CLASS

While there is no official definition of the middle class, most definitions depend heavily on an income classification. Households earning between $40,000 and $140,000 are usually viewed as middle class (Clark, 2001). The latest data available are categorized in a slightly different way, but still give a rough idea of how Latinos are doing with respect to this middle-class standard. Data from the 2008 American Community Survey are organized by quintiles with respect to household income, with the third quintile being $40,756–$65,176; the fourth, $65,177–$101,839; and the fifth, $101,839 and above. The percentage of Latino households that fall in the third and fourth quintiles combined is 38.4%, with only 11.6% falling into the fifth. This means that 50.1% of Latino households make more that $40,756, compared with 43.4% of Black, 63.9% of White, and 70% of Asian households. Perhaps the most striking comparison is within the fifth quintile; Blacks and Latinos respectively represent just 9.5% and 11.6% of households earning more than $101,839, while White and Asian households respectively represent 22.5% and 31.7% of this quintile within their racial groups (Pew Hispanic Center, 2010).

Some argue (Lowry & Michael, 1986, as cited in Clark, 2001) that income alone is not a sufficient measure of middle-class lifestyle, and suggest that incorporating home ownership into the definition is important. Of all households in which Latinos live, 49.1% are owner-occupied. By comparison, 45.8% of Black, 59.4% of Asian, and 73.4 % of White households are owner-occupied.

EDUCATION

As a group, Latinos age 25 and older are less likely than non-Latino Whites to have graduated from high school, at rates of 62.3% and 87.1%, respectively (U.S. Census Bureau, 2010b). Among non-Latino Whites, only 3.2% have less than a ninth-grade education, while 23.5% of Latinos fit this description. The statistics regarding completion of a college education are just as divergent. Only 13.3% of Latinos complete a bachelor's degree or higher, compared to 29.8% of non-Latino Whites (Pew Hispanic Center, 2010). There is also significant discrepancy in educational attainment within Latino groups; only 55.2% of Mexican origin individuals 25 years of age and older attained at least a high school education, compared with 76.4% of Puerto

Ricans and 80% of Cubans (U.S. Census Bureau, 2010b). Similarly, only 9.1% of Mexican origin individuals obtained a Bachelor's degree or higher, while 15.5% of Puerto Rican Americans and 28.1% of Cuban Americans obtained a Bachelor's degree or higher (U.S. Census Bureau, 2010b).

While graduating from college is an important achievement, it is increasingly difficult to develop into upwardly mobile and attain leadership positions across a variety of fields without an advanced degree. Of the 46.8 million Latinos in the U.S., only 935,000, less than 2%, have advanced degrees (U.S. Census Bureau, 2010a). Interestingly, while the mean earnings for Latinos increases from $44,696 for those with a Bachelor's degree to $84,512 for those with a professional degree, for non-Latino Whites, the increase is from $58,652 to $122,885. However, grouping White men and women together masks some significant differences across genders; White women earn significantly less at the bachelor's level ($42,846 vs. $73,477) and experience only a $40,000 increase with a professional degree, while White men experience a $70,000 increase (U.S. Census Bureau, 2010c).

CHAPTER 2

Sociopolitical History

INTRODUCTION

> Yo soy Joaquín,
> perdido en un mundo de confusión:
> I am Joaquín, lost in a world of confusion,
> caught up in the whirl of a gringo society,
> confused by the rules, scorned by attitudes,
> suppressed by manipulation, and destroyed by modern society (Gonzales, 1967)

For many of us, to be Latino in the United States is to know pain, to know struggle, to know discrimination and prejudice; perhaps beyond all, it is to know confusion, not just teenage angst as we search for personal identity, but a deeper, greater sense of confusion. It is a sense of perplexity, bewilderment, or disorientation. Even though it speaks primarily to the Chicano experience, nothing expresses this sense of confusion that many Latinos experience better and more succinctly than the poem *I Am Joaquín* by Rodolfo "Corky" Gonzales (1967). It is an epic poem well worth reading; presented at the start of the chapter is the beginning of the poem. It ends:

> I am the masses of my people and
> I refuse to be absorbed.
> I am Joaquín.
> The odds are great
> But my spirit is strong,
> My faith unbreakable,
> My blood is pure.
> I am Aztec prince and Christian Christ.
> I SHALL ENDURE!
> I WILL ENDURE!

To better understand and counsel Latinos, it is important to know their struggle; to know not only the very real struggle for physical survival but also the struggle for emotional, spiritual, and psychological survival, when more often than not we feel "scorned ... and destroyed" by the society in which we live. Some of you reading this book may very well know and have lived such a struggle. For those of you who have not, in this section of the book we offer you a glimpse of what that might be like; we will use excerpts from *I Am Joaquín* to more effectively portray that experience. This chapter is organized into two main sections. The first is a review of historical and sociopolitical factors that relate to all Latino groups. The second is divided into subsections that address issues specific to some Latino ethnic groups most heavily represented in the U.S.

COMMON HISTORY AND SOCIOPOLITICAL INFLUENCES

Ancestral Roots

Just as individuals must be viewed as products of their experiences, so must groups of people. The historical, sociological, political, and psychological foundations of present-day Latino communities have been influenced, to varying degrees, by three major cultural forces: Indigenous, Spanish, and African.

Latino Indigenous roots, as best we can figure, date back about 20,000 years to the last ice age (Ochoa 2001), when people from Siberia (Northeast Asia) walked across a solidly frozen Bering Strait and what is present-day Alaska. Because we later find evidence of thriving societies in Central and South America that date back to 7000 B.C., it is presumed that our original ancestors prospered and eventually worked their way south to those regions over the course of seven or eight thousand years. Societies rose, and declined to be replaced by new civilizations, so that by the time Christopher Columbus arrived in the "New World" in 1492, there were "Indigenous" communities in varying degrees of development all over the Western Hemisphere. Columbus's arrival serves as a convenient chronological marker because of the very significant changes that occurred in the hemisphere in the centuries that followed. Thus, we may speak of pre-Columbian civilizations or pre-Columbian cultures when we refer to our Indigenous roots. The three best-known pre-Colombian civilizations are the Aztecs in Mexico, the Maya in Mexico and Central America, and the Inca in South America. These well-established, flourishing, advanced civilizations had been in existence long before Columbus encountered the Western Hemisphere.

Although he was born in what is now Italy and lived in Portugal, Columbus arrived as an emissary of Spain. It was thus the Spaniards who played such a huge part in the history of the "New World" over the next several hundred years. The Spanish conquest may be viewed in positive terms ("the civilization" of the Western Hemisphere); it may be viewed in negative terms (the wanton destruction of Indigenous civilizations), or it may be viewed in neutral terms, as an example of humans repeating a history of conquest and empire building. They came and conquered, as they themselves had once been conquered. Unfortunately, in the process of conquering and taking for themselves the riches of the New World, the Spaniards decimated the native people through war, disease, and forced labor. Some authors suggest that as much as 96% of the native population perished (Carroll, 1991; Wade 1995); it is estimated, for example, that in Mexico there were 25 million people, of whom only one million remained after the conquest (Ochoa, 2001).

Africans entered the New World along with the first *conquistadores* in 1519. As the native population declined, Spaniards realized that they needed to bring in workers to replace the native populations, and Spanish governors in the New World literally begged the Spanish king to send slaves to the New World to provide labor in the mines, plantations, and textile factories already established there (Beltran, 1989). Over the course of the next hundred years, African slaves were brought in larger and larger numbers. By 1640, when the Portuguese slave trade to Spanish America was abolished (although it continued in other parts of the New World), New Spain (Mexico) contained the "second-largest population of enslaved Africans and the greatest number of free blacks in the Americas" (Bennett, 2003).

Spanish and African influence infused Indigenous cultures, a process somewhat analogous to the U.S. "melting pot" of European peoples. For several hundred years, Indigenous, Spanish, and African cultures mixed, mingled, and intertwined, and together they formed a solid foundation for what we now consider Latino culture. Much is written and known about the Spanish influences on Latino culture. In contrast, little is written, and even less has been formally researched, about Indigenous and African influences on Latino culture as we know it today. In our daily lives, however, we experience and know those influences. We know it in our music and our song, we smell it in our cooking, and taste it in our foods. We hear it, not in our formal Spanish language, but in the *caló* (slang) that rolls so easily off our tongues.

The First Latinos

In the sixteenth and seventeenth centuries, European males immigrated to the New World in large numbers, but European women did not readily follow. Thus, for hundreds of years, there were few European women present in Latin America, and few African women as well. Human biological drives being what they are, it is not surprising that European and African males would seek to have relations with (often unwilling) native women. It is fairly common knowledge that the leader of the first *conquistadores,* Hernán Cortés, was "given" a native "slave woman" (Malinche, baptized by a priest and given the name "Marina"). Malinche spoke two languages, Maya and Nahuatl, and she was given to Cortés to serve as his interpreter; to no one's surprise, she became his mistress (he was already married) and they had a son together. This son is considered the first *mestizo,* or person of mixed European and Indigenous descent: the first Latino (Lencheck, 1997).

In other parts of the New World, especially the Caribbean, where the Indigenous populations were completely wiped out and replaced by African slaves, the mixture with and sexual exploitation of African women by European males was more common, resulting in offspring called *mulattos.* In these areas, Africans made up 50% to 75% of the population, and by the end of the eighteenth century most Latin American societies included a significant population of descendants of Africans (Davis, 1995). By 1800, fewer than 20% of the population of the New World was of solely Spanish descent (Ochoa, 2001). Given this history, Latinos manifest phenotypical as well as sociological and cultural elements of three major groups: the Indigenous, European (Spanish), and African. As such, we Latinos range in skin color from white to black, and every shade in between. We have been master and slave. We are the conquerors and the conquered, and we are the oppressor and the oppressed.

> I am the Maya prince.
> I am Nezahualcóyotl, great leader of the Chichimecas.
> I am the sword and flame of Cortés the despot
> And I am the eagle and serpent of the Aztec civilization.
> I owned the land as far as the eye
> could see under the Crown of Spain,
> and I toiled on my Earth and gave my Indian sweat and blood
> for the Spanish master who ruled with tyranny over man and
> beast and all that he could trample
> But...THE GROUND WAS MINE.
> I was both tyrant and slave.

History of Oppression

In the first part of the sixteenth century, Spanish conquistadores invaded Mexico and Central and South America, killing and enslaving the Indigenous people. Enslaving people and exacting labor and goods from them was not new for the Indigenous people; the Aztecs had a society that included large numbers of slaves and commoners serving a small group of elite nobility. The Spaniards simply superimposed their feudal systems on an already existing structure. The Spanish king set up a system of viceroyalties and established firm royal control of all its holdings in the Western Hemisphere. From them, they exacted payments of gold and silver, which permitted Spain to become a great, rich, and powerful empire. In the New World, a few wealthy landowners dominated the economy. Where Indigenous populations had been wiped out, slavery was implemented and promulgated as part of the economy of the country. Two-and-a-half centuries after Columbus inadvertently landed on an island in the Caribbean, Latin America was completely controlled by a small group of European nations, of which Spain was the major player. The native people, the Africans, and their descendants were enslaved or forced to labor for minimal compensation by a few wealthy landowners and the Spanish crown.

If there are doubts that the history of domination and slavery affects Latinos to this day, one needs only to look at the language used by the people of Mexico and even people of Mexican origin in the U.S. In English, if a person does not hear what was said to him or her, the reply might be "excuse me?" or "what?"; in Mexican culture, it is not uncommon to hear the reply "*mande?*" in response to a statement or request that was not clearly understood. The word *mande* is a form of "*mandar*," which means "to command" or "to send." In essence, responding with "*mande?*" implies "command me," or "how can I be of service to you?," a response likely formed out of hundreds of years of servitude.

The Fight for Independence

Whenever and wherever slavery or oppression has existed, resistance eventually arises. It was no different in the New World; rebellions in the Caribbean, Mexico, and South America were myriad. The earliest uprising on record occurred in 1522 on a plantation belonging to Christopher Columbus's son Diego. In Mexico, slaves revolted in 1546, and in Venezuela, they rebelled in 1552 and again in 1556 (McKissack & McKissack, 1996). Beginning in the late eighteenth century and culminating in the early nineteenth century, however, the people of the New World rebelled almost en masse. One by one, the nations began severing their ties with the mother country, and by 1826 Spain had lost possession of all its New World territory except Cuba, which gained independence in 1898 at the end of the Spanish–American War, and Puerto Rico, which was absorbed into the United States at the same time. Unfortunately, the end of Spanish rule did not necessarily mean the end of oppression for most Latin American countries; as we will discuss in the following oppression, violence, and war would revisit Latin America often, greatly influencing U.S. Latino populations.

SPECIFIC LATINO ETHNIC SUBGROUPS

Previously, we focused on sociopolitical and historical factors common to all Latino groups. Despite these common factors, there are more differences among Latino groups than similarities, and some major political issues affect each group differently. For this reason, we have included this section, in which we provide greater detail on specific factors affecting each group.

Mexican Americans

Ethnic Labels

Like Latinos as a whole, people of Mexican descent in the U.S. have been called by many ethnic labels, including Mexican, Mexican American, Chicano, Hispano, Spanish, Spanish American, and Latin American. The term "Mexican American" will be used here, because we believe it to be the most inclusive and most widely accepted term for people born in the U.S. with ancestors from Mexico, although we will also use other terms if they serve to better describe the particular Mexican American group to which we are referring. We acknowledge that many individuals of Mexican origin in the U.S. are people who were born in Mexico, are citizens of Mexico, and may or may not be legal residents of the U.S. These individuals may not identify as Mexican American. Furthermore, it is important to understand the way issues, such as political consciousness and discrimination, affect self-labeling. "Chicano" is a politicized term, chosen by individuals of Mexican origin fighting for human rights causes—Brown Power—in the 1960s. Currently, labeling oneself "Chicano" does not necessarily mean identifying with those who are more cognizant of sociopolitical issues. Many Mexican American families who have resided in the United States for two or more generations identify as Chicano (Flores, Niemann, Romero, & Arredondo, & Rodriguez, 1999). However, for some Mexican Americans, the term, which originated from the derogatory slur "Mesheecano," retains its pejorative connotation from before its adoption by the Brown Power movement. While political solidarity may encourage people to embrace a label, discrimination can cause others to avoid certain terms. Guzmán, Keith, and Rico (2002) asked high school students of Mexican descent in central Texas about the way they self-labeled with respect to ethnicity. Some students, even those born in Mexico, talked about how they identified as "Hispanic" to distance themselves from the negative connotations associated with being labeled "Mexican." Niemann (2001) showed that stereotypes held by ethnic group members about themselves were very similar to the stereotypes held by out-group members about them. We discuss this experience in greater depth, and how it affects Latinos' mental health, in chapter five.

Presence in the United States

One of the unique characteristics of Mexican Americans is that parts of the present-day U.S. belonged to them at three or four different times in history. It belonged to their Indigenous ancestors (thousands of years ago), it belonged to their Spanish ancestors (five hundred years ago), and it belonged to their Mexican ancestors (two hundred years ago), and for those living in Texas, which was an independent nation for a short while, it belonged to their Texan or *Tejano* ancestors (170 years ago). Some politically conscious Mexicans and Mexican Americans say *"yo no cruce la raya; la raya me cruzo a mi,"* ("I did not cross the line; the line crossed me") or more accurately their ancestors; nonetheless, it connotes a certain attitude that they are not in the U.S. by choice but because it was imposed on them. Mexican Americans have had a very long-lasting significant presence in the U.S., and there is little doubt that they will continue to do so. By the terms of the Treaty of Guadalupe Hidalgo, which formally ended the Mexican-American War on February 2, 1848, all citizens of Mexico "residing within the ceded domain were to become citizens of the U.S. if they failed to leave within one year after the ratification of the treaty" (McWilliams, 1968, p. 51); less than two thousand people left within that timeframe. At the time, there were 75,000 to 80,000 Spanish-speaking people in the ceded territory. About 60,000 lived in New Mexico; another 7500 Spanish-speaking people lived in California; 5000 or so lived in Texas; and a few thousand lived in Arizona (McWilliams, 1968).

History of Oppression in the United States

Gold was discovered in California on January 24, 1848, just eight days before the Treaty of Guadalupe Hidalgo was signed. Word quickly spread about the discovery of gold, and people from the East rushed west in search of gold and to exploit the newly conquered lands. Thus, despite guarantees set forth by the Treaty, it did not take long for Mexican Americans to begin to feel the sting of oppression. "Anti-Mexican sentiment was ubiquitous throughout the Southwest" (Gonzales, 2000, p. 82), and violence was directed indiscriminately against native-born and immigrant people of Mexican descent. They were threatened or killed. Their legal rights were routinely ignored, and they were stripped of their land and possessions. Exploitation that could not be accomplished via threat of force was carried out via U.S. courts that sided with European-American plaintiffs. In the newly acquired land and in Texas, about 80% of Spanish and Mexican land grants were "legally" taken by Anglo-American lawyers and settlers (Ochoa, 2001). In Texas, entire communities were driven out of towns such as Austin, Seguin, and Uvalde. A mere six years after Texas gained its independence from Mexico, thirteen Anglo families owned 1.3 million acres of land; what was not "legally" taken with the help of land lawyers was taken by force. Violence against Mexicans was widespread; lynchings were common. The Texas Rangers, who were supposed to uphold the law, became a private security force for the powerful landowners. By 1870, tejanos, who a short time before had owned all of Texas, possessed only 10.6% of the wealth in Texas (Gonzalez, 2000).

The turn of the century did not make things better: abuses continued throughout the Southwest. The Texas Rangers were feared for the atrocities they committed; although held up as heroes and honorable men, "historically, no other police agency has evoked more fear, resentment, or distrust among Chicanos than the Texas Rangers. They represent the epitome of police abuse and brutality" (Mirandé, 1985, p. 75). Anyone who tried to defend himself or fight back was labeled a bandit and aggressively sought and killed. The Rangers "established a precedent, that is, whenever a suspect was arrested they would unceremoniously execute him on the road to Brownsville or to the jail, without giving him any opportunity. Frequently, we would find dead bodies and the ranches burned" (quoted in Martinez, 1996, p. 145). By 1920, "the Rio Grande Valley was as segregated as apartheid South Africa" (Gonzalez, 2000, p. 102). In Texas, "two separate cultural worlds—that of the Anglo-American and the Mexican—crystallized.... Language and culture placed Chicanos in conflict with the Anglo majority, which attempted to suppress their way of life. The Mexicans were considered aliens ... and they were intentionally denied control of their political, economic, and civil rights" (Acuña, 1972, p. 188).

During the middle of the twentieth century, the English-language media in California vilified young Mexicans and Mexican Americans, fabricating sensationalized stories of a Mexican "crime wave." Implicit in this maligning of Mexican American youth were also politicians, law enforcement, and social agency personnel who tended to perceive Mexican American youth as delinquent and violence-prone. This attitude culminated in the "zoot suit riots" of 1943, in which military personnel (sailors and marines) roamed the streets of Los Angeles seeking out and deliberately attacking Mexican American youth wearing the flashy outfits; these attacks "quickly extended to everyone who seemed to look like a Mexican" (Meier & Rivera, 1972), whether or not they were wearing a zoot suit. "For all intents and purposes, there was an undeclared war on Mexican Americans by roving packs of undisciplined servicemen.... To make matters worse, the shore patrol, city police, and the county sheriff's officials responded... [by] arresting the victims of the attacks rather than the attackers" (Meier & Rivera, 1972, p. 193).

Whether they are recent immigrants or whether their families have been in the U.S. for centuries, people of Mexican origin and their descendents have been treated as strangers in their own land. They have been threatened, chased off their land, cheated of their rights and possessions, and killed, and the perpetrators of such violence were rewarded and supported by legal and judicial authority. This is our legacy; it is a legacy that all historically and politically conscious Chicanos know and do not forget.

Migration Patterns

Migration patterns of Mexican people to the U.S. did not change much in the years immediately following ratification of the Treaty of Guadalupe Hidalgo. In the wake of the war, Mexicans continued to travel as they always had in search of opportunity or work or to be with family; what did change was that rather than simply traveling within their own home country, they were now traveling to a "foreign" country—the U.S. With the advent of the twentieth century came the "Great Migration" (1900–1930). This first wave of Mexican migration coincided with the "birth of the [U.S.] southwest as an economic empire" (McWilliams, 1968, p. 163) and with the political upheaval of the Revolution in Mexico. With these two push-pull factors at play, by the 1920s Mexicans became the dominant labor force in the mining and agricultural industries, especially after the advent of irrigation, which allowed the production of fruits, vegetables, and cotton to flourish in Texas and California (Gonzales, 2000). With the coming of World War I, there was an increased need for labor in other industries, resulting in the migration of Mexicans to industrial cities like Chicago, where they worked in the steel and automobile industries. The Great Migration ended during the Great Depression, but by that time, nearly 10% of the population of Mexico had crossed into the U.S., especially to the Southwest borderlands, where the population of Latinos of Mexican descent increased more than tenfold. By 1930, Los Angeles alone had over one million residents of Mexican origin. Only Mexico City and Guadalajara had greater numbers of Mexican people in a single metropolitan area (Gonzales & Gonzales, 2000).

The onset of World War II brought an increased need for labor in the U.S., prompting women to enter the labor force in record numbers. However, this was not sufficient to fill the increased need for industrial and agricultural labor. The U.S. found itself forced to look abroad for people to fill the great labor needs of a wartime economy (Durand, 2004). The most logical place to recruit workers was Mexico, and after a series of bilateral talks, the two countries reached an accord, the "*Bracero* Program," which sanctioned the use of temporary workers from Mexico, especially in agriculture and related employment (Meier & Rivera, 1972). Under the auspices of the Bracero Program, an estimated 4.6 million Mexican nationals migrated legally to the U.S. between 1942 and 1964 (Gutierrez, 1996). The workers returned to Mexico when their contracts expired, but one of the unanticipated effects of the program was that U.S. business owners became aware of a readily available Mexican labor force that could be exploited. At the same time, people from Mexico learned that there was plenty of work to be had by a person willing and able to work for wages which, though low, were better than those available in Mexico. Since that time, the economies of both the U.S. and Mexico have influenced the ebb and flow of migration from that country, and the experience set the stage for a steady flow of legal and illegal migration that to this day seems all but unstoppable. Annual migration from Mexico increased from about 450,000 in the 1960s to 650,000 in the 1970s, and jumped to 1,650,000 in the last two decades of the twentieth century. Furthermore, not only did the influx of Mexican immigrants continue in the traditional locations (the Southwest and major industrial cites) but they are also now flooding into new destinations all over the country, places such as Tennessee, the Carolinas, Minnesota, and Georgia (Grieco, 2003). As we will discuss in Chapter 3, illegal immigration and the proposed solutions to this dilemma have been, and will continue to be, a hotly debated topic in the twenty-first century.

Repatriation

While U.S. business owners profit from the availability of a cheap labor force, the society as a whole has never greeted immigrants from Mexico very warmly. Just like there are patterns of increased immigration, there have been patterns of "repatriation," usually forced. When the U.S. economy is growing, there is a greater need for Mexican labor, but when there is recession and high unemployment rates, people become concerned that Mexicans may be taking jobs that could benefit U.S. citizens, and there is increased pressure on the U.S. government to deal with the "Mexican problem" (Gonzales, 2000). The government usually responds by "repatriation," a euphemism for deporting "illegal" or undocumented workers. There are three types of "repatriates": those who leave voluntarily, those who succumb to scare tactics or threats of deportation and leave, and those deported by immigration officials (Meier & and Rivera, 1972; Gonzales, 2000). The first repatriations occurred in 1931, shortly after the Great Depression began; the largest numbers of repatriations occurred in Texas (an estimated 132,000) and California (between 50,000 and 75,000). It is estimated that over 400,000 Mexican people were repatriated during the Great Depression, as many as half involuntarily and some illegally (Meier & Rivera, 1972; Gonzalez, 2000).

After the Korean War, a recession again led to fears that Mexicans were taking scarce jobs from U.S. citizens, and "Operation Wetback" was formally instituted on June 1954 (Garcia & Greigo, 1996); the U.S. government sanctioned brutal dragnets conducted in hundreds of Mexican neighborhoods. Immigrants were summarily arrested and thrown in jail, then herded into trucks or trains and deported. Many of those deported were U.S. citizens, but the government ignored all due process and deported between one and two million Latinos of Mexican descent in a few months (Gonzalez, 2000). As soon as the recession ended, however, the *Bracero* program was reinstituted, and Mexicans were once again not only welcomed but also enticed to come into the U.S.—to await the next economic downturn when they would be maligned and deported once again.

Puerto Ricans

Puerto Ricans, the second-largest Latino group, are U.S. citizens; thus rather than being immigrants as are many other Latinos, Puerto Ricans are migrants, and are free to travel back and forth from the island to the U.S. mainland without restrictions. Their travel from Puerto Rico to or within the U.S. is akin to any U.S. citizen traveling from one state to another. This arrangement began in 1917, when the island ceased to be a U.S. territory and became a Commonwealth. The issue of whether Puerto Rico should remain a Commonwealth or instead become a state is one that periodically comes up in referendum votes, but maintaining Commonwealth status has received the majority of support up to this point (Santiago-Rivera, Arredondo, & Gallardo-Cooper, 2002). The struggle over this issue reflects the struggle for national identity.

Puerto Rico poses for us, as a nation, our greatest shame and our greatest pride. For more than five hundred years, the history of Puerto Rico has been the history of colonial oppression. From the landing of Christopher Columbus, the decimation of the Taíno natives, the repopulation with African slaves, four hundred years of Spanish rule, to a century of U.S. colonialism, Puerto Rico is the story of "uninterrupted colonial bondage" (Flores, 1993, p. 111). It is our shame that we continue to hold a nation in bondage; it is our pride that the Puerto Rican spirit is indomitable. Puerto Rico and its people are a microcosm—the essence—of American-ness in the broadest sense of the word: the "Western Hemisphere."

It is the knowing of Puerto Rican culture and national identity that is the greatest challenge for the student of Latino culture. As a people, the Puerto Ricans have struggled, as do many Latinos, to find their identity and establish their nationhood. In that struggle, they have confronted and debated their own class, racial, gender, and national prejudices. Puerto Ricans are a "Nation on the Move." "It is an elusive culture, half hidden in the past and only half-seen in the present" (Duany, 2002), and it is full of apparent contradictions that can only be understood if one understands the racial history of Puerto Rico. Rodriguez (1996, p. 25) explains:

> The experience of Puerto Ricans ... points more clearly than any researched materials to the chasm that exists between Whites and Blacks in the U.S. and the racism that afflicts both groups. For within the U.S. perspective, Puerto Ricans, racially speaking, belong to both groups; however, ethnically, they belong to neither. Thus placed, Puerto Ricans find themselves caught between two polarities and at a dialectical distance from both. Puerto Ricans are between white and black; Puerto Ricans are neither white nor black.

The Puerto Rican culture is based on and reflects, perhaps more than any other, the three main roots of the cultures of the Americas: Indigenous, European, and African (Duany, 2002). The Puerto Rican community is the model of Latinidad in the U.S., the struggle of living, breathing, negotiating, and being two identities at once. In this section, we will attempt to familiarize you with that struggle.

Ethnic, Racial, and National Identity

Ethnically, Puerto Ricans may identify with any of the following ethnic labels: Puerto Rican, *puertorriqueño,* U.S. Puerto Ricans, Boricuas, and *Borinqueños* (the last two derived from the aboriginal name for the island). For Puerto Ricans living in New York City, terms such as "New York Puerto Rican, Newyorican, Neorican, Nuyorican, *nuyorriqueño,* or simply Rican" have also been adopted.

Like Mexican Americans, Puerto Ricans continue to struggle mightily with the issue of national identity. The process of establishing a solid sense of national identity has been complicated significantly by two main questions: racial identity and political identity. Political identity is the struggle related to the political relationship between the U.S. and Puerto Rico. Puerto Rico is a U.S. "commonwealth" or *estado asosiado libre*. It is another contradiction in the Puerto Rican experience. Puerto Rico is and is not part of the U.S. It is a confusing political relationship and a divisive issue for Puerto Ricans, as they are about equally split in the desire to remain a commonwealth and to become a state. In 1993, the issue was put to popular vote; 48.6% of voters opted for Puerto Rico to remain a commonwealth while 46.3% voted to seek statehood. In 1998, another vote resulted in very similar results; 50% favored continuing commonwealth status and 47% favored statehood (Schaefer, 2002). Puerto Ricans continue in a 90-year-old state of limbo. They have American citizenship but without full rights; Puerto Ricans are subject to the military draft and are eligible for government-sponsored assistance programs, but do not pay federal income tax and cannot vote in U.S. elections.

The issue of racial identification is a deep and emotional issue; for many years, Spanish or European roots were strongly emphasized or viewed with a greater sense of pride than Indigenous or African roots. This appears to be changing, however, and Puerto Ricans are starting to recognize and accept the very significant contribution of their African and Indigenous ancestors, and now the "American" (U.S.) influence. The racial identity issue becomes more complicated for Puerto Ricans born and/or raised on the U.S. mainland, primarily in the New York City area. The racial and ethnic classification system and attitudes in Puerto Rico, and in other Latin American countries, are more flexible than those of the mainland U.S. The racial classification system in the U.S., a socially constructed system designed to advantage some over others, is based on phenotype (facial features and hair texture) and skin color. However, instead of seeing color on a continuum, the old "one-drop" rule still seems to influence racial categorization. That is, if you appear Black, you are seen racially as Black. The system is rigidly "either/or." Puerto Rico uses a classification system based on phenotype and skin color, but the categorization system is more fluid, and may also take into account social class and other social meanings related to race, which allows for a "spectrum of racial types" (Rodriguez, 1996). Racial categories may be as descriptive and creative as saying someone is the color of "*café con leche*", which literally means "coffee with milk", and is meant to describe someone with light brown skin. In Puerto Rico, there is also more acceptance of social intermingling of people of different color and racial characteristics (Fitzpatrick, 1987).

When Puerto Ricans first arrived in New York, they experienced a significant culture shock, as the vast majority of Puerto Ricans have some degree of African ancestry and were thus treated with the same disregard, prejudice, discrimination, and hostility as mainland-born African Americans. The angst of this experience is poignantly described by Piri Thomas (1967) in his autobiographical novel *Down These Mean Streets*. Born of Puerto Rican and Cuban parents, Piri is born the *negrito* (dark-skinned) of the family, while his siblings are born *blanco* (white). Growing up in Spanish Harlem during the Great Depression, he spends his late teenage years and young adulthood trying to make sense of his cultural and racial experience. He's not black, but "Nothing falls right" with "*los Blancos.*" One day he tells his brother José, "I'm a Negro," and his brother counters, "No, you're a Puerto Rican." The discussion leads to a heated argument and then a physical altercation, after which Piri tells his father, "[José], you, and James think you're white, and I'm the only one that's found out I'm not. I tried hard not to find out. But I did.... Poppa ... what's wrong with not being white? ... I'm black and it don't make no difference whether I say good-bye or *adiós*—it means the same.... I'm proud to be Puerto Rican, but being Puerto Rican don't make the color" (p. 147). After a long struggle with himself and others that included a seven-year stint in prison, Piri comes out of the experience without having really resolved the Black and White question, but having gained some self-acceptance.

This experience was common for many darker-skinned Puerto Ricans growing up in New York in the 1950s, 1960s, and 1970s, and like Piri, many reached a point of self-awareness and self-acceptance that they were, as Rodriguez stated, "between white and black ... [and] neither white nor black." Ironically, this self-realization was that they were not only neither White nor Black but also that they were not exactly Puerto Rican either, and they self-identified using new labels, such as those mentioned earlier: Newyorican, Neorican, Nuyorican, and nuyorriqueño. In sum, the issue of self-identification for this group, ethnically, nationally, and racially, is still unsettled; in this monograph, however, we will primarily use the term "Puerto Rican," although at times we might use one of the other terms, such as "Nuyorican," if it serves as a better or more accurate descriptor of the population at issue.

Presence in the United States

During the eighteenth century, there was a flourishing trade between the U.S. and Puerto Ricans, who at the time were subjects of the Spanish Crown; there is little doubt that Puerto Ricans entered the mainland U.S. during that time. The first official record of a Puerto Rican immigrating to the U.S. was that of Eugenio María de Hostos, a journalist, philosopher, and freedom fighter, who arrived in 1874. He had been instrumental in a rebellion against Spain known as *El Grito de Lares*. When this attempt to liberate Puerto Rico from Spain failed, de Hostos and other freedom fighters were exiled and came to New York. Thus began a small community of Puerto Ricans in New York City, which over the course of the next century would grow to over a million people. Furthermore, Puerto Ricans would disperse across the U.S., settling in all fifty states and forming vibrant communities in major metropolitan areas like Chicago, Miami, Los Angeles, and Houston.

History of Oppression in the United States

The U.S. took possession of the island of Puerto Rico in 1898 after the Spanish-American War. Being a commonwealth, during the first half of the twentieth century, the U.S. president appointed the governor of Puerto Rico, and even today the Puerto Ricans on the island do not control monetary or military policy (Weaver, 1994). One hundred years of economic policy set by the U.S. government has resulted in Puerto Rico having an overall economy that is well below that of the poorest areas in the U.S. (Alicea, 1994; Schaefer, 2002). Puerto Ricans on the mainland do not fare much better. They are the most economically disadvantaged Latino group in the U.S., and their poverty rate is three times the national average. Their communities in urban areas are plagued with problems such as poor educational opportunity and attainment, high crime rates and drug use, high unemployment, and breakdown of the family structure (Green, 2000). In addition to the institutionalized oppression just discussed, Puerto Ricans have faced individual discrimination and prejudice for over a century. As indicated earlier, because of their African ancestry many Puerto Ricans on the mainland have been subjected to the same type of oppression and discrimination as African Americans. Furthermore, they have been discriminated against in jobs, housing, and education because of their Spanish language (Sanchez, 1993), a situation which persists to this day.

Migration and Settlement Patterns

Puerto Ricans began migrating to the U.S. almost immediately after the island was declared a U.S. territory. Though not great in number, the flow of migrants leaving the island was steady, and it is estimated that between 1920 and 1930 some 52,000 Puerto Ricans lived in other parts of the U.S. Fortyfive states reported the presence of Puerto Rican migrants, who traveled as far away as California and Hawaii, where they worked harvesting crops (Korrol, 1994). The largest wave of migrants, however, came in the decade after World War II. The era is referred to as the "Great Migration," and it is estimated that the number of Puerto Ricans on the mainland increased from about 70,000 to 301,000 by 1950, and they could be found in all states of the union. Economic conditions on the island never improved, and migration to the mainland continued at a rapid pace. The number of Puerto Ricans in the U.S. more than doubled between 1950 and 1960, when 887,662 were counted by the census. By 1970, that number had increased to 1.4 million, and to 3.2 million by 1990. The 2000 census counted 3.4 million people of Puerto Rican heritage on the U.S. mainland, predominantly concentrated in the northeastern states, and 3.8 million on the island. According to the U.S. Census, the states with the largest Puerto Rican populations in 2000 were New York, Florida, New Jersey, Pennsylvania, and Massachusetts. The latest data show 4.1 million people of Puerto Rican descent living in the U.S. (Pew Hispanic Center, 2010).

Cubans

Cubans are the third-largest Latino group in the U.S. Cuba and Puerto Rico have similar histories; both were occupied by Spaniards who entirely wiped out the Indigenous population and subsequently brought slaves from Africa to repopulate the islands. Furthermore, because of the "sugar revolution" which started in the late eighteenth century, there was a tremendous need for labor in Cuba, and Africans were brought en masse late in the colonial period. By the mid-nineteenth century, African slaves accounted for 44% of the population. Because by that time the interest of the Spanish was wealth rather than "civilization," there was no effort to acculturate the Africans into Cuban Spanish society. This made "the continued vitality of many elements of African culture" in Cuba possible, in sharp contrast to other colonial states (Grenier & Pérez, 2003). By the end of the nineteenth century, in Cuba there were hundreds of thousands of first- or second-generation Africans, whose culture was primarily rooted in African rather than Spanish traditions. In spite of African culture being a major aspect of Cuban society, immigrants to the U.S. were drawn not from the poorer, African segment of the population, but rather from the more affluent, "Whiter" portion of Cuban society, a fact that has played a major role in the experience of Cuban immigrants and their descendents. Grenier and Pérez (p. 37) go as far as to suggest that "many Cubans in the U.S. are second and third generation Spaniards," and more than 90% of the Cubans in the U.S. identify as White.

Ethnic Labels

Cubans possess a strong insular identity that is independent of any developing Hispanic or Latino sense of identity. Grenier and Pérez (2003) report that a bumper sticker seen in Miami proclaims, "I am not Hispanic, I am Cuban." People from Cuba and their descendents do not commonly self-identify as Cuban American, but rather as *Cubano/a,* or as Cubans. In this monograph we will use these two terms interchangeably. For Cubans, the issue of ethnic label or identification has not been as important or as prominent in personality development as has been the "exile perspective." The exile mentality dominated the Cuban experience in the U.S. during the nineteenth and twentieth centuries, and continues to be an issue into the twenty-first century. The vast majority of Cubans who immigrated to the U.S. did not do so by choice, but by circumstance. For most immigrants, there are pull factors from the country they are entering. For Cubans, emigration has been forced upon them by push factors in Cuba, primarily fear for their lives and the safety of their families. Given these circumstances, first-generation Cubans have always hoped to return to Cuba when it is safe to do so. Consequently, they have resisted identification as "immigrants," preferring to think of themselves as "exiles," and the "exile character ... played a central role in forming community identity and defining the nature of Cuban integration into North American society" (Poyo & Díaz-Miranda, 1994). What has been created in the U.S., however, is a "Cuba-in-exile." In essence, Cuban exiles tried to recreate life in the U.S. as it had been in Cuba, and indeed, south Florida today is often called "little Havana" or "Havana, USA." Cuba, however, is a very different country today than it was fifty years ago, and what Cubans have created in south Florida may be unrecognizable to inhabitants of modern-day Cuba.

Presence in the United States

Historically, Cubans have had a presence in the U.S. since 1560, when St. Augustine, Florida was established (Poyo and Díaz-Miranda 1994). They started coming in large numbers in the early nineteenth century, and they have come for two main reasons: in search of political stability and of economic opportunity (García, 1996). Félix Varela is considered to be the first

Cuban to immigrate to the U.S., in 1823. Varela entered the U.S. after fleeing from Spain, where he was persecuted for seeking Cuban freedom from the mother country, and as such his arrival marks not only the beginning of Cuban history in the U.S., but also "established the tradition of Cuban political exile in the U.S." (Grenier & Pérez, p. 16).

In the 1830s, Cuban cigar factory owners relocated to Key West, Florida in order to avoid high U.S. tariffs on their products (Alicea, 1994). Cubanos were not a significant presence in the U.S., however, until the latter part of 1860's, when approximately 100,000 Cubans sought refuge from war in Cuba and settled in Florida and the northeast (New York, Philadelphia, and Boston). By the 1880s, Cubans had established social, economic, and political power in Florida, particularly Key West; so much so that in 1876 a Cuban was elected mayor of that city, and other Cubans were elected to county and state offices. After the turn of the century, as a consequence of the end of Spanish rule over Cuba, World War I, and the Great Depression, Cuban immigration decreased, and by 1930 the presence of Cuban-born persons in the U.S. had actually declined. By mid-century, there were still some "well-defined Cuban communities" in various parts of the U.S., especially New York and Florida, but whereas in the late 1800s the number of Cuban-born individuals in the U.S. had exceeded the hundred thousand mark, and by 1959 that number totaled only about forty thousand.

Migration and Settlement Patterns

In 1959, Fidel Castro and his followers defeated the dictator Fulgencio Batista and established a socialist regime in Cuba. That year marks the beginning of an exodus that has brought over three quarters of a million Cuban-born people into the U.S. It has been, in the words of Grenier and Pérez (2003, p. 20–21), "one of the longest-running human dramas on the world stage. A seemingly interminable saga that has spanned more than forty years and continues into the 21st century." Since 1959, the arrival of Cuban-born people in the U.S. happened in four dramatic, clearly defined episodes. Between 1959 and 1962, approximately 200,000 persons arrived, including about 14,000 children without parents; these first arrivals were labeled the "Golden Exiles," because overrepresented in his group were the "Cuban elite" or upper class. The vast majority of these new arrivals settled in Dade County, Florida. Between 1965 and 1973, the Cuban government permitted relatives of the Golden Exiles to leave Cuba. This started in 1965 as a boatlift (five thousand left in boats), but was quickly suspended, and subsequently Cubans were only allowed to leave by airplane. These are the "freedom flights" which brought approximately 260,000 Cuban-born people into the U.S. Since these immigrants were relatives of the early Golden Exiles, they naturally settled in Dade County with their families. In April 1980, the Cuban government announced that "all Cubans who wished to leave the island would be permitted to do so and urged them to call their relatives in the U.S. to come pick them up" (García, 1996, p. 60). For five months, Cuban exiles in the U.S. boarded their boats and navigated 90 miles of ocean from Florida to the port of Mariel in Cuba to pick up their relatives. In those five months, 125,000 Cubans entered the U.S. Again, a majority of them settled in Dade County, Florida. This exodus was termed the "Mariel

Boatlift." The next wave of Cubans entered the U.S. in 1994. In August of that year, the Cuban government announced that it would not try to detain anyone attempting to leave Cuba. In a desperate attempt to escape, thousands of people launched themselves into the ocean on rafts or other makeshift, unseaworthy vessels. The U.S. Coast Guard rescued close to thirty-seven thousand people within a month (Grenier & Pérez, 2003). The rescued rafters were taken to the U.S. Marine base in Guantánamo, where they were detained for over a year before being admitted to the U.S.

As we come to the close of the first decade of the twenty-first century, about 1.6 million *Cubanos* live in the U.S.; 979,490 (60.1%) are Cuban-born and the majority live in southern Florida, particularly Dade County and the Miami metropolitan area (Pew Hispanic Center, 2010). Cuban communities, however, may be found throughout the U.S. Larger communities are found in the Northeast, especially New York, New Jersey, and Connecticut, and smaller communities exist in states like California, Texas, and Illinois (Ochoa, 2001).

History of Oppression in the United States

Cubans, especially those entering after 1959, have been given special status as political refugees and privileges that other Latino groups have not received (Grenier & Pérez). There are several reasons for this, the main one being strong U.S. sentiment against Fidel Castro and his socialist/communist regime. In addition, as a society, we have been much more accepting of immigrants from European or upper- or middle-class backgrounds. Cuban immigrants who entered the U.S. in the first and second wave (the Golden Exiles and the Freedom Flights) fit neatly into these categories; about 97% were White and middle or upper class (García 1996). They were well received and special accommodations were made to facilitate their success and integration, if not assimilation, into U.S. society. García (1996) notes that the financial assistance offered to Cubans in Florida in 1960 was significantly greater than that offered to local citizens. Cubans were also the first group to receive government-surplus food (the service was later extended to state and local agencies), and in Florida, job training and English instruction programs were established for Cubans, something not available to local citizens. This is not to say that Cubans did not experience oppression and discrimination; "No Cubans Allowed" signs were seen, and many local residents expressed their displeasure with the new immigrants (García, 1996). In addition, the Cubans from the Mariel Boatlift (the *marielitos*) and the rafters included people other than the Cuban White middle- and upper-class elite. The *marielitos* were predominately male, about 20% were Black or Mulatto (of mixed Black and White heritage), over half of them did not have family or friends in the U.S., and most were working-class people. These immigrants were not received with open arms as their predecessors had been. Furthermore, the *marielitos* were not viewed as "legitimate refugees," and therefore did not qualify for the federal assistance program from which earlier Cuban immigrants had benefited. This third wave of Cubans were "the most stigmatized group of immigrants in recent history" (García, 2003, p. 70). There was public outcry about their acceptance in Florida and the rest of the U.S.; public opinion held that Castro had opened the doors of prisons and mental institutions and sent us Cuba's undesirables. Thousands of immigrants from the third and fourth waves were placed in detention facilities or "resettlement camps." They were not allowed to leave and remained confined for extended periods of time while "sponsors" could be located. The majority of the camp residents were single Black or Mulatto men who could not easily get sponsors. The term, *marielitos,* took on pejorative connotations, and several riots at a resettlement camp in Fort Chaffee, Arkansas worsened the image problem. The press picked up the story and subsequently there were a series of articles commenting about the "criminal environment" that had developed in the camps. In Miami, those who were released from resettlement camps without appropriate sponsorship roamed the streets.. They perpetrated many crimes; over a third of Miami's murders in 1980 were committed by *marielitos.* As the U.S. government began to look more closely at the background of the *marielitos,* they found that many of the new immigrants had histories of criminal behavior and mental illness, and they were placed on a list of "excludables." In 1985, in exchange for an agreement to accept twenty thousand legal immigrants from Cuba, the Cuban government agreed to take back 2,746 detainees of the Mariel boatlift, but this never came to full fruition (García, 1996), and many remained indefinitely detained. It took prison riots, a lot of public consciousness, several court battles, and about a dozen years, but eventually all the *marielitos* who were detained were released into U.S. Cuban communities (about 1600) or deported to Cuba (about 400).

By the time the *marielito* crisis was over, the untainted image of Cubans that had been created by the remarkable success of the Golden Exiles had been badly tarnished, and as early as November 1980, anti-Cuban sentiment was strong and would remain so for many years. In part, it was this sentiment that led to unsympathetic views of the next wave of Cuban immigrants, the rafters or *balseros.* In a reversal of a three-decade long policy, Cubans picked up at sea by the U.S. Coast Guard were no longer brought to the U.S. but rather were taken to the U.S. naval base in Guantánamo with the expectation that they would remain there until they were accepted by a third country or returned to Cuba. This did not stop the *balseros,* and before long there were seventeen thousand people awaiting their fortune in Guantánamo. This crisis ended when, once again, the U.S. agreed to accept twenty thousand legal Cuban immigrants annually in exchange for the Cuban government restricting illegal migration. However, in addition to this legal immigration policy, an "illegal" immigration policy remains in place. Currently, any Cuban attempting to enter the country who is intercepted by the U.S. coastguard before touching U.S. soil is returned to Cuba, but Cubans who touch U.S. soil before being apprehended are granted permanent residency.

Repatriation

Because of the U.S. policy toward Cuba and the Castro regime in particular, repatriation has not been an option for Cuban immigrants. As indicated previously, during times of crisis Cuban immigration has been supported, and at times promoted, by the U.S. government. Although Fidel Castro has retired from government, and his brother Raúl succeeded him as President in February 2008, he still remains a prominent figure in Cuban politics, and the country remains under communist rule ("Raúl Castro named Cuban president," 2008). A half-century after the Golden Exiles came to the U.S., Castro's legacy endures, and the first Cubans still remain, as their name clearly suggests, in exile. As far as is known, only about four hundred Cubans have been repatriated; they were primarily Cubans who entered the U.S. during the Mariel Boatlift and who were later identified as "excludables."

In spite of, or perhaps because of, their tenacious hold on their exile identity (and rejection of an immigrant identity), Cubans in the U.S. have managed to become one of the most successful immigrant groups in the U.S. Both exile communities (pre-Cuba Libre and post-1959) were politically and economically successful. They adjusted well to U.S. society while retaining a very strong sense of ethnic identity, never losing sight of the goal of recovering their homeland. It has given them a "strong singular identity" that sets them apart from other immigrant and Latino groups (Grenier & Pérez, 2003).

OTHER LATINO GROUPS IN THE U.S.

After the three largest Latino groups just discussed, the next largest percentage of Latinos in the U.S. are the 1.7 million reporting their origin as "Other Spanish/Hispanic/Latino." Following that group are the 1.5 million people of Salvadoran descent and 1.3 million of Dominican background (Pew Hispanic Center, 2010). All the other Latino groups have less than a million each, but that is not to say that they do not have a significant presence in many states around the country. Because Latino immigrants often go to places where they have family or where there is a critical mass of people from their home countries and cities, even smaller numbers of Latinos can begin to shape communities across the U.S.

Dominicans

The original inhabitants of the island on which the Dominican Republic is located were long ago decimated by European enslavement and disease, and a new society was formed. Thus, as far as nations go, the Dominican Republic is a new nation, and in some ways, it is still developing its national character. The same is true for Dominican Americans; they are relatively new to the U.S. scene, and are attempting to find their place in this country. Similarly, we the receiving country seem to know little about the Dominican Republic and its people, and we find ourselves with many misconceptions about them. For example, we do not know that they are a highly educated, professional, proud, and independent group.

According to Ricourt (2002), there are "three different, yet interconnected identities in the Dominican community": new immigrants, established Dominicans, and Dominican Americans. These identities are affected by many variables, including migration status, employment, length of residency in the U.S., and location, but one primary variable is the continuous migration of new immigrants from the Dominican Republic to the U.S.; this "affects how Dominicans engage in the process of identity formation" (Ricourt, p. 15). The new immigrant's ethnic identity is "rooted in the homeland." The established Dominicans have a dual identity that may include a longing to return to the homeland while being well established in the U.S.; they may even have dual citizenship. Finally, Dominican Americans include both established immigrants and second-generation Dominicans. They may visit the homeland, but they do not long to live there. Like the established Dominicans, the ethnic identity of Dominican Americans may still be somewhat fluid. Ricourt states that some Dominican Americans are struggling with the angst and search for identity common to second-generation immigrants.

History of Oppression in the United States

In the Dominican Republic, socially derived categorizations (family of origin, education, and economic status) are more pronounced than the racial categorization of Black, White, or Mulatto (Hendricks, 1974). Furthermore, in Dominican society "to be partly White is to be non-Black," so most Dominicans consider themselves White (Pessar, 1995, p. 43). It is a rude awakening for most Dominicans who come to the U.S. to find the opposite view. Here they are considered Black based on the color of their skin, irrespective of origin, education, or economic status, and they experience the full force of discrimination experienced by African Americans in the U.S. (Pessar). They find themselves being rejected for jobs because of the color of their skin, and they also experience the same prejudice as African Americans in the media and the institutionalized racism inherent at the local, state, and national levels.

In a study conducted by Itzigsohn, Giorguli, and Vazquez, (2005), 418 Dominicans were asked about their racial identification. Interestingly, when asked how they defined themselves racially, the largest categories were: Hispano/a (21.1%), White (2.9%), and Black (5%), with other categories like *Indio/a* (10%) and *Dominicano/a* (9.8%) receiving more endorsement than "White" and "Black." However, when asked "How do you think mainstream Americans categorize you racially?" the answers were Hispano/a (29.4%), White (6.2%), and Black (35.6%). This demonstrates not only the flexibility of racial categorization in the Dominican Republic but also the awareness that in the U.S. the majority of Dominicans may be categorized as Blacks and treated accordingly.

Migration and Settlement Patterns

The Dominican Republic has had close political and economic ties to the U.S. for many years but migration to the U.S. is a relatively recent phenomenon, dating back about forty years to the early 1960s. Prior to 1962, the restrictive government of Rafael Trujillo had limited migration to the U.S. When that government was overthrown, a "mass exodus" to the U.S. began almost immediately. During the 1960s, about 11,500 Dominicans emigrated to the U.S. each year; the number rose to 16,000 annually during the 1970s, and in the 1980s over 30,000 Dominicans entered the U.S. each year

(Ochoa, 2001). In fact, the Dominican Republic is the nation that sent the most immigrants to New York City during the last three decades of the twentieth century (Ricourt 2002). The population of Dominicans nearly doubled from 1990 to 2000, from approximately 348,00 to 687,000 foreign-born (Grieco, 2004), making Dominicans one of the fastest growing immigrant populations in the U.S.

As suggested here, the earliest migrations were politically motivated. There was significant political unrest in the Dominican Republic, and the U.S. (who had a military presence on the island at the time) created a "safety valve" to alleviate unrest. They started issuing visas, and emigration soared from about one thousand to about ten thousand per year. Like the Cuban exiles, the first wave of Dominican emigrants was comprised of middle- and upper-class people who feared for their safety. Later, the Dominican Republic saw not only some political stability but also economic disaster. The salary differential between the U.S. and the Dominican Republic went from 4:1 in 1980 to 13:1 by 1991. Coupled with high unemployment rates, this created intense push factors, and migration became driven by the necessity to search for economic opportunity (Pessar & Graham, 2001).

Most Dominicans enter the U.S. legally, although some overstay their visa and subsequently become "illegal." As is true of some Mexicans, Dominicans may pay $2,000.00 to $5,000.00 and risk their lives to be brought in illegally by a *coyote*. Whether they enter the U.S. legally or illegally, most Dominicans take advantage of the *cadena* (chain or link) of kinship or friendships in order to facilitate their arrival and subsequent success. Many Dominicans already in the U.S. feel obligated to assist newcomers, and according to Pessar (1995, p. 19), "it would be virtually inconceivable for established immigrants to request that a relative or close friend reside in a commercial establishment or alone during the initial period of settlement." It is of course anticipated that one would eventually pay back the assistance, either in kind or in monetary remuneration. In any case, the cadena promotes migration to areas where family or friends are already established, promoting the settlement of new Dominican immigrants in established Dominican communities. As a result, most Dominicans are clustered in a few states in the Northeast (80.3%), the majority (52.4%) in New York. Other states with significant Dominican populations include New Jersey, Massachusetts, Pennsylvania, and Florida (Pew Hispanic Center, 2009).

Central Americans

Central America is comprised of seven independent nations: Belize, Costa Rica, El Salvador, Guatemala, Honduras, Nicaragua, and Panama, representing a richly diverse mixture of cultures. Most Central Americans speak Spanish, but English is the official language of Belize and is also widely spoken on the Atlantic coast of Nicaragua. In addition, many native tongues are still spoken throughout the region; in Guatemala alone, more than twenty distinct native languages survive and are spoken daily; about 40% of the population speaks one of four major Indigenous languages: Quiche, Mam, Cakchiquel, or Kekchi (Hong, 2000).

The peoples of Central America include Indigenous peoples, Europeans, Africans, and mestizos (Hernandez, 2004), although percentages vary. Costa Rica, for example, is populated primarily by White people of European descent; they constitute 96% of the population (Chase, 2000). By contrast, 89% of Hondurans are mestizo, as are the majority of people in Panama and El Salvador, while the Maya still predominate in Guatemala. Catholicism is the primary religion in most Central American nations, but in Guatemala it is strongly influenced by Mayan traditions. In Guatemala, Pentecostal Protestants have made strong headway, and about a third of Guatemalans practice some form of this denomination (Hong, 2000).

The countries also have different political histories. Belize, for example, only became an independent nation in September 1981, more than 150 years after the other nations declared and gained independence from Europe. Perhaps it was this fact that protected Belize from the political unrest and civil wars experienced by the other Central American countries, with the exception of Costa Rica. In comparison to the rest of Central America, Costa Rica has maintained egalitarian and democratic ideals and enjoyed a stable government and economy since it became a sovereign nation in 1838.

Ethnic Labels

Central America is an ethnically and culturally diverse region between Mexico and South America, and although they share much, each of the seven nations has its own rich history. Perhaps because of their similarities to other Latino groups and because they are relative newcomers, Central Americans have not been the focus of specific discrimination and stereotyping by the mainstream population, but they suffer the same discrimination and stereotyping that is directed at Latinos in general. Central Americans, like other immigrants to the U.S., are proud of their national heritage, and because they frequently settle in "friendly communities," they have the opportunity to continue practicing and celebrating their ethnic differences, both in the community at large and in their homes (Hernandez, 2004). As with many other Latinos, Central Americans prefer not to be labeled with pan-ethnic terms such as "Hispanic" or "Latino," and even a less inclusive term like "Central American" or *Centroamericano* may be too broad when speaking about immigrants from Central America. There is a world of difference in the lived experience and reasons for migration between an English-speaking immigrant from Belize and a Mayan from Guatemala. The term "Central American" lacks utility, and using labels that specify national origin—such as *Salvadoreño, Hondureño,* Guatemalan, or *Guatemalteco*—is most useful when discussing Central American immigrants. Like many other Latinos, Central Americans eschew pan-ethnic labels, and even though they may acknowledge their connection to this country, be it by birth or citizenship, their ethnic identity remains firmly rooted in their national origin (Ramos, 2004).

United States Political Involvement in Central America

U.S. involvement in Central America dates back to the drafting of the Monroe Doctrine in 1823, when the U.S. established its policy of "having the right to prevent expansion of European Power in the Western Hemisphere." Subsequently, in 1840 U.S. businesses begin investing in Central America, opening mines and growing crops like coffee and bananas, and by the early 1900s the U.S. Navy was conducting routine patrols of the Caribbean Central American coast, "protecting American lives and property in port towns" (Ochoa, 2001, p. 119). In the early part of the twentieth century, American interference in Central America escalated from patrolling the coast to military action and the invasion and occupation of Central American countries including Nicaragua, Honduras, El Salvador, Guatemala, Costa Rica, and Panama. By the mid-twentieth century, U.S. foreign policy in Central America included outright approval and support of oligarchies and dictatorships, as well as military backing for the overthrow of democratically-elected presidents. During the cold war period and its aftermath, and as "a direct result of military and economic intervention by our own [U.S.] government" (Gonzalez, 2000, p. 129), Central American countries experienced a period of dramatic social instability, marked by "military dictatorships, right-wing death squads, guerilla insurgencies, poverty, and hunger" (Novas, 1998, p. 233).

Presence in the United States

Central American immigrants, although not large in number, have had a presence in this country for close to two centuries; however, their numbers were relatively small in comparison to other Latino groups until the last quarter of the twentieth century (Hernandez, 2004). As other immigrants have done, Central Americans have tended to flock to large cities and neighborhoods where they have family or friends. Costa Ricans and Panamanians represented the largest Central American groups for decades, although this would change in the latter part of the twentieth century. New York and Los Angeles have always attracted new immigrants, and it has been no different for Central Americans, although Chicago also had well-established Central American communities before immigration began en masse. One Salvadoran community in Chicago dates back to the 1920s. Panamanians have been in New York since the last century, and arrived in Chicago shortly after World War II as brides of American servicemen who had been stationed in the Canal Zone (Smagula, 2000).

History of Oppression in the United States

With the exception of Costa Ricans, the vast majority of Central Americans are mestizos or Indigenous peoples, and therefore similar to Mexicans in body type and skin tone. This, and the fact that Central Americans were for many years a very small percentage of the Latino immigrant population, meant that mainstream U.S. society either overlooked them or lumped together with other Latino groups. As a result, there is little history of discrimination or stereotyping of Central Americans specifically, although they certainly suffered the discrimination, prejudice, and strong anti-immigrant sentiment that was—and continues to be—levelled against all Latino groups. This is particularly true for the large number of undocumented Central American immigrants, who are denied basic human rights, thereby facilitating their abuse and exploitation.

Furthermore, the U.S. government discriminated against Guatemalans, Salvadorans, and Hondurans, refusing to grant them political asylum, even though they were doing so for well over 50% of Nicaraguan immigrants. As a result, all undocumented immigrants are relegated to work clandestinely, always fearing discovery and job loss, as well as being vulnerable to unscrupulous employers who deny them pay for their hard work.

Migration and Settlement Patterns

During the nineteenth century, the number of Central Americans legally entering the U.S. was small, averaging less than one thousand per decade (Hernandez, 2004). During the first few decades of the twentieth century, the number increased dramatically to about sixteen thousand between 1921 and 1930. The number decreased to about six thousand between 1931 and 1940, but increased again in the 1940s to about twenty thousand. Subsequently, as the political unrest, described previously, began to unfold, the number of Central Americans entering the United States began to increase significantly. About 45,000 entered in the 1950s; that number doubled to 100,000 in the 1960s, and continued to increase as the situation, or "*la crisis,*" worsened in Central America. In the 1980s, about twenty-five thousand Central Americans legally entered the U.S. each year. Official records indicate that between 1980 and 2000 about a million people left Central America and legally entered and settled in the U.S. It is estimated, however, that another 470,000 are here without proper documentation (Hernandez, 2004). Pew Hispanic Center data (Suro, 2002) suggest that official records may reflect an undercount of as much as 680,000. Currently, there are approximately 3.8 million Central Americans living in the U.S (Pew Hispanic Center, 2008).

Central Americans risk life and limb to come here. Migrants making the 2,500-mile trek from Central America to the U.S. risk robbery, rape, enslavement, and death, only to arrive in the U.S. as undocumented immigrants to be treated like criminals. They are considered to be in the U.S. illegally, and they are always subject to apprehension and deportation.

Today, Central America is more stable, but widespread poverty still exists, prompting people from the region to continue to migrate. It is important to note that about 88% of the Central Americans in the U.S. come from four countries: El Salvador, Guatemala, Honduras, and Nicaragua. Recent immigration data continue to reflect a similar pattern of migration; between 1990 and 1999, immigrants from these four countries accounted for about 90% of the total legal immigration from Central America (Office of Immigration Statistics, 2009). Salvadorans are the largest of the Central American immigrant groups, comprising about 41% of all persons of Central American origin in the U.S., followed by Guatemalans (25%), Hondurans (15%), and Nicaraguans (9%) (Hagan and Rodriguez, 1996; Pew Hispanic Center, 2010).

South Americans

South America is comprised of thirteen countries, many of which have very little in common (Barnett, 2004). Nine of the thirteen countries are Spanish-speaking, and therefore Latino, nations: Argentina, Bolivia, Chile, Columbia, Ecuador,

Paraguay, Peru, Uruguay, and Venezuela. Even though these countries share a common language, there are significant historical and cultural differences among them. Argentina, for example, is 85% White and has more in common with European nations than with its Latin American neighbors. In contrast, Peru and Ecuador are about 80% mestizo or Amerindian, and continue to hold fast to Indigenous traditions.

South American immigration to the U.S. in significant numbers is a recent trend, prompted by economic and political problems for which the U.S. is partly responsible (Barnett, 2004; Gonzalez, 2000; Novas, 1998).

> [During the Cold War the] United States frequently supported corrupt Latin American regimes—even brutal dictators—in order to protect its own economic and strategic interests in the region…. For the United States, preventing the Soviet Union from gaining a foothold in the Western Hemisphere was of paramount importance. Thus, American policymakers were willing to support even the most repressive and corrupt Latin American regimes as long as they were anti-communist (Barnett, 2004, p. 21).

Four decades of this type of U.S. policy and interference significantly hindered democratic, economic, and social development in South America, promoting instead political destabilization and economic chaos in the region and providing significant push factors for migration. Some countries saw as much as 20% of their population displaced, usually to neighboring countries, but a significant percentage migrated as far north as the U.S. and Canada.

Ethnic Labels

South Americans are a diverse group of people, and they have a long history of competing and even fighting with one another (Ochoa, 2001). On the other hand, South American nations have often been compassionate, helpful, and cooperative during times of crisis. This was especially true in the latter part of the twentieth century, when political refugees from troubled countries simply crossed over to safety in a neighboring country. Their fierce independence, national pride, and distinct cultural backgrounds make it difficult for them to identify as a group, however, and there does not seem to be an appropriately inclusive term to use, except perhaps "South American." Latino does not fit those who identify with their Indigenous roots, and Hispanic cannot truly be applied to Whites of Italian, German, Irish, Jewish, or other non-Spanish ancestry. Thus, as with Central Americans, when referring to individual South American immigrants it is best to use the term associated with their nationality, such as *Colombiano, Argentino,* or *Peruano.*

The U.S. Census Bureau started reporting separate records for individual South American nations in the 1960s. Available data suggest that since that time, all South American groups have shown a similar pattern of rapid increase from 1960 to 1990, such that by the turn of the century the 100,000 South Americans counted in 1960 had increased to about 1,350,000. The latest figures show about 2.7 million South Americans living in the U.S (Pew Hispanic Center, 2010).

History of Oppression in the United States

Given the diversity of the South American population, the manner in which South American immigrants are received and treated varies significantly. The more "European" immigrants, such as Argentineans, tend to experience less discrimination; the same is true for better-educated immigrants, especially if they have a good command of the English language. Colombians are often labeled as "drug-dealers," or as somehow having connections to or benefiting from drug money, especially if they are financially successful. Some immigrants have experienced "in-group" discrimination by other Latinos because they speak a "different Spanish" than the community at large; this is especially true for Argentineans who use "vos" instead of "tu." Mestizos or darker-skinned immigrants are lumped together with other Latino groups and may experience stereotyping as "Mexicans" and thereby suffer the prejudice and discrimination levelled against members of that group. There have not been any repatriation movements targeting South Americans since 1849, but deportations are common. Countless numbers of highly educated professionals have their educational degrees and professional experience completely discounted because their credentials are not accepted in the U.S., and doctors and university professors may be relegated to washing dishes for a living.

CHAPTER 3

Current Issues

MENTAL HEALTH RISKS

Accessibility and Adequacy of Healthcare
Poverty and Lack of Insurance

A number of factors contribute to inadequate healthcare for Latinos, chief among these are lack of education and financial resources. As discussed in Chapter 2, Latinos lag behind at all levels of education, make less money than Whites, and have a higher proportion of poverty in comparison to the United States population overall. Lower levels of education lead to higher unemployment, lower-paying jobs, and lack of benefits (or less generous benefits) which in turn contribute to a lack of adequate healthcare services (Ruiz, 2002). We know that poorer benefit and health insurance packages can mean less choice in the selection of doctors and other healthcare professionals, less support for receiving second opinions, less direct access to specialists, and less coverage for long-term health issues. Even with some insurance, lower income may mean an inability to pay deductibles and co-pays.

In 2008 the percentage of Latinos who lacked health insurance was 31.7%, down from 32.1% in 2007 (U.S. Census Bureau, 2010). Again, the comparison with non-Latino Whites is striking, with only 10.7% of this group being uninsured. For Black Americans, the uninsured rate is 19%. However, grouping native- and foreign-born Latinos together masks an important discrepancy. At 20.4%, native-born Latinos have an uninsured rate similar to Blacks, but foreign-born Latinos have an alarmingly high uninsured rate of 50.1% (Pew Hispanic Center, 2010).

While there are many community agencies that do a valiant job of serving the neediest Latinos, they are often overwhelmed by clients, which may lead to long waits for evaluations or therapy appointments. Finally, while we are avid supporters of allowing supervised counselors-in-training to treat clients in community mental health settings, this means both that Latino clients are often receiving services from the least experienced therapists in the field, and that student therapists are being asked to take on extremely challenging cases in which Latino clients may present with multifaceted issues. While there may be shortcomings to public mental health, one of the advantages is location, if the center happens to be located in or near a Latino neighborhood. Unfortunately, there is a lack of clinics, hospitals, and other mental health facilities located in Latino communities or accessible by public transportation. This situation acts as a major barrier to accessing treatment (Vega & Lopez, 2001).

Under-Representation of Latinos among Mental Healthcare Professionals

While Latinos currently represent about 15.4% of the total population in the U.S., only 5.4% of physicians, 4.6% of psychiatrists, 3% of nurses, and 1% of psychologists are Latinos (Dingfelder, 2005; Ruiz, 2002). This makes for a small number of people in the healthcare and mental healthcare professions who can relate on a personal level to Latino culture. This also means that Latino clients are unlikely to see someone who looks like them—or who they perceive will understand them—when they seek help for physical or emotional ailments. For this reason, it is especially important to support education in the Latino community and to see that educational institutions at all levels commit to creating environments that value Latino culture, and attract and retain Latino students.

If you are a healthcare professional and not Latino, there are steps you can take to increase your cultural competency and better serve your Latino clients. First and foremost, educate yourself about Latino culture. If you are reading this book then you are already taking the first step. Secondly, learn Spanish, to whatever extent is realistically possible in your situation. We concede that becoming fluent in another language is difficult when the process is started in adulthood, but even a rudimentary command of Spanish will help in connecting with and treating Latino clients. Finally, seek supervision or consultation if you think you may not be in a position to adequately meet the needs of Latino clients.

Language Issues

Often, a lack of Latino healthcare providers also means a shortage of bilingual administrative and treatment staff. This issue also contributes to Latinos receiving less mental healthcare. Upon examining the use of the public mental health system by Latinos in California for the period from mid-year 1997 to mid-year 1998, Vega and Lopez (2001) reported that rates varied widely among counties. For instance, Los Angeles County, with a greater availability of bilingual staff and an urban location, had a proportionately higher use rate than Fresno County, which contains both urban and rural areas and had low numbers of bilingual service providers.

When Latinos do access the mental health care system, language barriers often lead to misdiagnosis. This occurs most frequently with Spanish-speaking

Latinos and English-speaking clinicians. However, this may also occur with Latinos who do speak English, but who may conceptualize their illness differently from therapists and doctors with different worldviews (See Chapter 4). When Spanish-speaking Latinos are interviewed by clinicians in English, misunderstandings occur regarding the presence of symptoms and the frequency, duration, and severity of those symptoms. This may lead to misdiagnosis (conceptualizing the illness incorrectly), underdiagnosis, or as has been reported in the literature, "an exaggerated perception of psychopathology" (Ruiz, 2002, p. 86). We might expect that the use of interpreters would alleviate such issues, but often it does not, and this type of assistance is fraught with its own challenges.

Use of Interpreters

It might be expected that the use of interpreters would alleviate some of the issues described in the previous section, but often it does not, and this type of assistance is fraught with its own challenges. Interpreters who are not trained in psychology or mental health issues may not accurately translate a clinician's query or the client's response. Furthermore, if a friend, family member, or someone else invested in the client's situation is used, information may be either misrepresented or misinterpreted, intentionally or unintentionally, to steer diagnosis toward a certain outcome. Using children as interpreters is especially problematic, as a family structure in traditional Latino families tends to be hierarchical, wherein children would not be expected to have intimate knowledge of their parents' difficulties, nor would they be in a position to "speak for" their parents regarding such matters. Also, cognitively, children cannot be expected to decipher and translate a clinician's questions in the same manner as an adult. In June, 2005 the California State Assembly approved a bill to prohibit the use of children under the age of 15 as interpreters in hospitals, clinics, and doctors' offices (Keigwin, 2005). Clearly, this is a serious issue that has attracted the attention of both lawmakers and society at large , and its practice constitutes at the very least lack of ethical practice by medical and mental healthcare providers.

Racism and Discrimination Stressors
Influence of Stereotypes

In an article focused specifically on Latinos of Mexican descent, Niemann (2001) discussed the unfortunate fact that many individuals of Mexican origin hold the same stereotypes about themselves as do certain members of White mainstream society. These stereotypes include being lazy, uneducated, inferior, and irresponsible. Along with this, Niemann proposes that stereotypes may become prescriptive rather than merely descriptive, meaning that Latinos begin to believe these stereotypes to be true of themselves and shape their behaviors and choices to conform to these societal expectations, even if they are negative. This process is known as *internalized oppression*, and it has very negative implications for one's mental health. This type of thinking can be seen in Latino adolescents who say that they do not want to study or do well in school, because it is a "White" behavior, or who reject their fellow Latinos who do succeed academically, calling them "sell-outs." They have come to believe that academic success is not for them, that perhaps they are not capable of it, and that it is incompatible with their ethnic identity. Unfortunately, internalized oppression is often reinforced by individual, institutional, and cultural racism.[1] In a review of selected studies conducted between 1965 and 2000, Williams and Williams-Morris (2000) found positive associations between internalized racism and lower self-esteem, chronic health problems, and depression in people of color and other targeted groups.

Racist Incidents as Trauma

While "racist incidents" may call to mind images of violent crimes such as the James Byrd murder in 1998, they also include nonviolent and quite current examples such as a Latino teen being suspended from school in Kansas City in December 2005 for speaking Spanish. However, day-to-day "mini-traumas" continue to impact the lives of Latinos and other people of color (Bryant-Davis & Ocampo, 2005, p. 483). Sue and colleagues defined these incidents, which they termed "microaggressions," as "... brief, everyday exchanges that send denigrating messages to people of color because they belong to a racial minority group. [They] are often unconsciously delivered in the form of subtle snubs or dismissive looks, gestures, and tones" (Sue et al., 2007, p. 273).

Examples of microaggressions include: a U.S.-born Latino being told he speaks "good English," or an assumption being made that such a Latino speaks Spanish; a well-educated Latina being told "You're a credit to your race" or being referred to as an "exception"; or a Latino man mowing his own lawn being asked how much he charges. There are also incidents of discrimination in which Latinos are denied access or opportunity or may have their rights restricted, such as being denied promotions or a mortgage, or being pulled over for a traffic violation. While we may not think of these situations as "traumatizing," they may be for some individuals.

The *Diagnostic and Statistical Manual of Mental Disorders* (4th ed., text revision; *DSM-IV-TR*; American Psychiatric Association, 2000) has a limited scope in that it conceptualizes trauma only as physical in nature (injury, death, or threats of these). Bryant-Davis and Ocampo (2005) examined the parallels between racist experiences and acknowledged traumas such as rape and domestic violence. The authors propose that symptoms such as denial, shock, dissociation, and self-destructive behaviors can be seen in some survivors of racist events just as they are seen in many survivors of rape and domestic violence. The authors note limitations to the parallel model, but their main point stands: "Counselors should address the traumas of societal

---

[1] Carter (1997) proposes three levels of racism: *Individual*, one who has come to accept without question, consciously or subconsciously, the societal messages that people of color are inferior to Whites; *Institutional*, laws, customs, and practices which systematically reflect and produce intentionally and unintentionally racial inequalities in American society; and *Cultural*, the conscious or subconscious conviction that White European American cultural patterns or practices are superior to those of other visible racial or ethnic groups.

oppression with the concern and compassion that are afforded survivors of other traumatic experiences" (p. 495). Studies found positive relationships between discrimination and psychological distress in Latinos (Amaro, Russo, & Johnson, 1987; Finch, Kolody, & Vega, 2000; Salgado de Snyder, 1987, as cited in Williams & Williams-Morris, 2000; Williams, Neighbors, & Jackson, 2003).

Stress and Trauma of Crossing the Border

For those Latinos who come without documents from Mexico and Central and South America, crossing into the U.S. is a mental health risk in itself. Cubans, and sometimes Dominicans, also face some of the issues that will be discussed here, but instead of dealing with the dangers of a land crossing, they face the risk of drowning due to overcrowded or less-than-seaworthy boats. Whereas Mexican individuals must cross one border into the U.S., Central and South Americans must cross multiple borders. Unfortunately, all Latinos who enter the U.S. illegally are criminalized for seeking the opportunities for survival and success that many of us, who are U.S. residents and citizens, often take for granted.

Crossing the border holds many dangers. Many people pay guides or *coyotes* thousands of dollars to get them across, and these individuals sometimes take advantage of vulnerable immigrants, take their money, and leave them to fend for themselves in the desert. There is the risk of dying of dehydration, starvation, heat stroke, or being murdered by drug traffickers or other criminals. Women live in constant fear of being raped. Sometimes, immigrants are held captive against their will after arriving in the U.S. if relatives are unable to pay the guides. The National Human Rights Commission reported that 1600 migrants are being kidnapped in Mexico every month (Dvorak, 2010) and that border violence has increased since 2008, when the drug cartel war in Mexico began (Borunda, 2010). In August 2010, seventy-two migrants traveling to find work in the U.S. were murdered by the henchmen of one drug cartel (Dvorak, 2010). Even if a migrant arrives safely, there is a constant fear of being deported. Hiding, being on the run, or living a life where one must constantly be "on the lookout" creates chronic anxiety that can be both mentally and physically debilitating. Unfortunately, the fear of being reported and deported keeps people from seeking services. Children who cross the border face all the same dangers as adults, but there may also be confusion about why the journey is being undertaken.

In many instances, parents who cross the border into the U.S. must leave their children behind. The emotional stresses that accompany such a decision are multiple. There is guilt for leaving children and other family members behind and constant concern for their well-being. These parents may experience sadness or depression at not being able to see their children on a regular basis. The children grow up with an absent father or mother, and the relationship with the parents may become distant or estranged. The children may experience anger, fear, or anxiety about being left behind, as well as abandonment issues that follow them into future relationships.

Latino Immigrant Backlash

If individuals do survive the crossing, there are still many obstacles to face. There is the powerlessness and limitations in opportunity that come with being undocumented, such as being restricted to the low-paying and/or long-hour jobs available to those without papers or with fake documents. There is also the trauma of crossing. Immigrants may develop post-traumatic stress disorder (PTSD) due to rape, assault, or other near-death experiences. Due to a lack of resources, these individuals are often relegated to low-SES, high-crime neighborhoods where children are exposed to drugs, prostitution, or other criminal activity. If they are able to live with family members who are already established in the U.S., the situation may be slightly better, but then there may be issues of overcrowding, limited privacy, and conflict due to more than one family occupying the same household.

Acculturation challenges, which will be further discussed in Chapter 4, include a new language, different cultural norms, and the need to make new connections. For children, there is a new school, an unfamiliar educational system, and new friends. Since "different" is often interpreted as "deficient" (Ogbu, 1987), children may be ostracized for their lack of English, different foods in their lunch, and other conditions that may come with a lower SES status, such as old or worn clothing.

In addition to these challenges is the immigrant backlash that appears to have reached a new level of vitriol in the first decade of the twenty-first century. This can manifest itself through anti-immigrant hate crimes such as those reported in Suffolk County, NY, where seven high school students fatally stabbed an Ecuadorean immigrant in 2008; teenagers torched a house because "Mexicans lived there" in 2003; and two white men stabbed and beat two Mexican day laborers in 2000 (Southern Poverty Law Center, 2010). The FBI reported that between 2003 and 2007, anti-Latino hate crime violence rose 40% nationwide (Southern Poverty Law Center, 2010). On the other end of the spectrum are the legal maneuvers that are being instituted to target Latino immigrants, such as a 2008 ordinance passed in Farmer's Branch, Texas, attempting to regulate the residence of noncitizens within its borders, but found unconstitutional by a federal judge (MALDEF, 2010), and SB 1070 passed in Arizona in July 2010 that requires police to demand papers from people they stop who they suspect are "unlawfully present" (MALDEF, 2010). The Mexican American Legal Defense and Education Fund (MALDEF) is challenging the Arizona law. While these crimes and laws may target undocumented Latinos, they evoke anger, stress, and frustration, and create an unwelcoming and hostile atmosphere for all Latinos.

CONTEMPORARY ISSUES AND IMPLICATIONS FOR MENTAL HEALTH

Mental Health in Latinos

A report by the U.S. Department of Health and Human Services (2001) found that Latino youth are at a "significantly higher risk for poor mental health outcomes." They are more likely to report depression, drop out of school, and experience suicidal ideation than their European American peers. There have been mixed findings regarding the prevalence of depression among Latinos as compared to European Americans, with some studies reporting higher rates among Latinos, and others stating the opposite (Beltran, 2005). These discrepancies may be due to differing methodology, such as the instruments used to measure depression.

The phenomenon known as the *immigrant paradox* has been documented extensively in the literature with respect to Latinos and healthcare outcomes (Alegría et al., 2008). For Latinos, having spent less time in the U.S. and being less acculturated (i.e. primarily speaking Spanish and engaging in Latino cultural practices) has been related to a host of positive health behaviors, such as a lower likelihood of consuming fast-food, a lower likelihood of using drugs and alcohol, and a greater likelihood to adhere to prescribed health regimens (Allen et al., 2008; Unger et al., 2004; Mainous, Diaz, and Geesey, 2008). This immigrant paradox appears to hold with respect to mental health issues as well.

Latino immigrants tend to have lower rates of psychiatric disorders than U.S.-born Latinos. However, rates of disorders in immigrants increase over time, especially for those who arrived as children (Vega & Lopez, 2001; U.S. Department of Health and Human Services, 2001). Conversely, Latinos born in the U.S. or who have spent a considerable amount of time in the U.S. are more likely to be diagnosed with psychiatric disorders than are foreign-born or more recently arrived Latinos (Alegría et al., 2008). For recent immigrants, the increase in disorders over time may be largely attributable to the stressful process of having to adapt to a new location, language, customs, and values, but it may be due to increased and prolonged exposure to racial microaggressions, racial discrimination and their negative consequences as described earlier in this chapter. As immigrants learn that the American dream may not be accessible to them after all, disillusionment may turn to anxiety, depression, and other emotional and physical disorders. Over generations, the oppression faced by Latinos and other people of color is often internalized.

However, this connection between acculturation and health outcomes has recently been questioned. Because acculturation has often been measured simplistically and unidimensionally (see Chapter 4 for a discussion of acculturation models), it is unclear if the immigrant paradox may be due to the loss of native culture practices or if it is due to acquiring the practices of the receiving culture (Schwartz, 2010).

Post-Traumatic Stress Disorder (PTSD) in Latinos

Pole, Best, Metzler, and Marmar (2005) present evidence, including their own findings, that Latinos in the U.S. have higher rates of PTSD than non-Latino Whites and non-Latino Black Americans. These differences were found in police officers, residents of New York City who experienced the September 11th terrorist attacks, victims of Hurricane Andrew, and combat veterans (Pole et al., 2001; Perilla, Norris, & Lavizzo, 2002; Galea et al., 2002; Kulka et al., 1990, as cited in Pole et al., 2005) Pole et al. found that Latinos experienced more dissociation immediately after traumatic events, were more likely to underreport distress, had greater avoidance and numbing after these events, and used passive coping to deal with the aftermath of the trauma. The authors connect these behaviors to cultural norms including the tendency to be stoic, to keep problems in the family, to be fatalistic (reliance on faith, a higher power, luck, or daydreaming to improve the situation), and the common presence of dissociative symptoms in Latino "culture-bound" syndromes. While much more research is needed, Pole et al. (2005) call on therapists to be aware of the higher PTSD rates among Latinos and to understand how cultural factors may play a role in this phenomenon.

Psychological Distress in Gay and Bisexual Latino Men

For reasons to be discussed in Chapter 4, gay, lesbian, and bisexual Latinos are in need of a great deal of support due to the complex layers of discrimination they face from society, other Latinos, and their own families. Diaz, Ayala, Bein, Henne, and Marin, (2001) found higher rates of distress, including anxiety, depressed mood, and suicidal ideation, in a sample ($N = 912$) of self-identified gay and bisexual Latino men drawn from three cities in the U.S. These authors attribute these mental health difficulties to the social alienation and low self-esteem that result from living in an oppressive environment.

INTEGRATED HEALTH CARE

There is a growing body of evidence that demonstrates that integrating physical and behavioral health care has positive health benefits (Hogg Foundation for Mental Health, 2010a). Most of the time, individuals see a primary care physician in one location and seek mental health treatment in another, a situation which can lead to uncoordinated and ineffective care. Due to transportation issues or the cost of co-pays at each location, people may only make it to one place or the other. On the provider's side, there is the issue of test results, diagnosis, and medication information being situated in more than one chart, and releases having to be signed on each side for any information sharing to occur. One approach to integrating physical and behavioral health care is the "collaborative care" model, which places a primary care physician and a mental health professional at the same site to improve care. This model has four essential components: a mental health assessment instrument that screens clients for mental health issues; a clinical care manager, a professional or paraprofessional who works with mental health consumers in the primary care setting, and monitors their response to treatment; a patient database used to coordinate patient information; and a psychiatrist who supervises the clinical care manager and makes recommendations for medication. The clinical care manager focuses on mental health treatment and providing psycho-educational information to consumers and their families, but does not coordinate social services needs (Hogg Foundation for Mental Health, 2010b).

In 2006 the Hogg Foundation for Mental Health launched a $2.6 million, three-year grant program to bring the "collaborative care" model of integrated health care to several clinics in Texas (Hogg Foundation for Mental

Health, 2010a). As a recipient of the grant program, Project Vida Community Health Clinic in El Paso used their funding to add mental health services to their existing physical care programs (Kristo, 2009). In addition to the integrated care model, the clinic is a wonderful demonstration of cultural competency with respect to serving the Latino community, with murals of children's art decorating the walls and women in traditional Mexican dresses dancing to Latino music in the community room alongside women and children participating in art therapy.

> Doctors glide in and out of medical exam rooms, in between visits by "promotoras," community health workers who also phone clients to ask how they're doing or why they missed their weekly nutrition class. First names are used. Family members are inquired about. The meaning of "cultural competency" becomes apparent here, where staff and medical professionals blend and become one with the largely Mexican-American population they serve (Kristo, 2009).

While integrated healthcare is powerful in and of itself, the Project Vida sample demonstrates how much more effective great healthcare innovations can be when paired with cultural competency.

HEALTH CARE REFORM

The Patient Protection and Affordable Care Act (PPACA) is a federal statute that was signed into law in the United States by President Barack Obama on March 23, 2010. Together with the Health Care and Education Reconciliation Act of 2010 (signed into law on March 30, 2010), the Act is the product of the health care reform agenda of the Democratic 111th Congress and the Obama administration, and is now referred as the "Affordable Care Act" (Wikipedia, 2010). The law allows for a number of health-related provisions to come into effect over a period of four years, including the expansion of Medicaid eligibility, insurance premium subsidies, incentives for businesses to provide health care benefits, the prohibition of denial of coverage/claims based on pre-existing conditions, the establishment of health insurance exchanges, and support for medical research. However, the benefits of these changes for Latinos remain to be seen.

The health care reform plans do not provide for the coverage of undocumented immigrants, of whom 59% are uninsured, nor would it cover legal immigrants who are in their first five years of residency in the U.S. (Marrero, 2009). However, the Affordable Health Care Act is said to focus on many of the issues that prevent Latinos from achieving better health, such as access to good healthcare, by providing support for community health centers that serve low-income populations, new training requirements for medical professionals, and loan and scholarship programs to encourage these professionals to practice in underserved communities (Pecquet, 2010). The White House has set up a Spanish-language version of its HealthCare.gov insurance portal (www.CuidadoDeSalud.gov) in order to highlight the benefits of the reform for Latinos (Pecquet, 2010).

STRESSORS OF THE RISING LATINO MIDDLE CLASS

The majority of this chapter focuses on issues that affect Latinos who are poor, undocumented, or otherwise have limited resources. It is worth mentioning that as some Latinos do attain more education and higher incomes, they begin to face a number of issues that may impact their mental health, such as the stress of dual-earner couples. As Latinas move out of the traditional gender role of the stay-at-home mother, they may face the stress of continuing to try to fulfill the ideal mother role, maintain a household, and manage a career. The complementary side of this issue is Latinos who are more open to partners who work outside the home and who are more willing to take on household responsibilities. Both sides of this equation weigh on the mental health of those trying to negotiate these new gender roles. For Latinos who choose a non-Latino partner, there are the difficulties of negotiating cultural differences in the relationship and between the families, and there may be the challenge of raising biracial and bi-ethnic children.

While home ownership is a privilege that only half of Latinos have, paying a mortgage and maintaining a home can be stressful as well. The financial crisis that began in 2008 saw many home foreclosures. Because most Latinos do not have a long legacy of educational access and financial security, they may not have as much experience in financial matters such as managing credit or investing. Finally, "success" for many Latinos means working at a level in an organization where there are few other Latinos. This may bring the stress of feeling like you cannot be yourself, or cannot bring the Latino parts of yourself to work. We talk more about ethnic identity development in Chapter 4. While Latinos with more limited resources will certainly face a host of mental health challenges and barriers to treatment, it is important to remember that educated and financially better-off Latinos face unique challenges as well.

Cultural Systems

INTRODUCTION

Understanding how Latino clients make sense of their ethnic and racial group membership and their world, and which values drive their actions, choices, and decisions will allow you to better understand them as a people and to design interventions that will be both appropriate and effective. While there are a number of factors that are important to consider in understanding Latinos, in this chapter we address some of the core issues of identity, specifically those of ethnic and racial identity development. These two separate processes are discussed from the perspective of academic models designed to help us understand their components, as well as from the personal stories of both authors. Various impacts of the acculturation process on Latinos are also discussed, including changing gender roles, language issues, and parenting challenges. You will also be introduced to the broad concepts of worldview and cultural scripts, followed by a discussion of more specific Latino cultural values and how they may interact with counseling interventions. Throughout the chapter, you are cautioned to consider that Latinos will differ in their adherence to the cultural norms being presented here depending on their generation, level of acculturation, and other demographic factors. Finally, we will examine areas of resiliency and strength that are often not given enough recognition in discussions of the mental health challenges faced by Latinos.

ETHNIC IDENTITY

While it cannot be assumed that race and ethnicity are the most salient identities for any individual Latino or person of color, we can say with some certainty that mainstream society will initially react to these aspects of a

Latino's identity, because they are visible. Furthermore, we would argue that all people—Latinos, people of color, and White European Americans—go through a developmental process in which they make sense of their ethnic and racial group memberships, but that individuals are in different phases of this process at different points in their lives. For these reasons, we think it is important to introduce you to the models of ethnic and racial identity development and to discuss how you might address these issues in your work with clients.

We can learn about people from diverse cultures through scholarship, but it is only through personal relationships that we can truly know them. We started a personal relationship with you by way of our short biographical statements presented at the opening of this text and through discussing ethnic identity development, and we will deepen that relationship as we write about our own experiences, thoughts, and struggles with this process. For each of us, the search for and development of our ethnic identities has been a struggle. Ethnic identity development concerns making sense of your ethnic group membership and figuring out how you uniquely and personally experience being a part of your ethnic group. Each individual must figure out this process for himself or herself, and there are no "right" answers or conclusions to this exploration process. Neither is there a definite endpoint, as our identities continue to develop over a lifetime. In order to know Latinos it is crucial to understand the process and struggle surrounding ethnic identity development.

Ethnic identity can be thought of as the process of being socialized into one's own ethnic group (Casas & Pytluck, 1995). Ethnic identity, as conceptualized by Phinney (1990, 1992), involves a sense of belonging to your ethnic group (affirmation), an interest in finding out about the traditions of that group (exploration), and an awareness of the role that ethnicity will play in your life (achievement). This last concept, that of resolving and internalizing the meaning of your ethnicity for your life, has also been conceptualized in the literature as "resolution" (Umaña-Taylor, Yazedjian, & Bámaca-Gómez, 2004). Phinney (1996) outlined three stages of ethnic identity development: unexamined, during which ethnicity is not a salient part of the self-concept, and there is an acceptance of the attitudes and values present in the person's environment; exploration, a time during which interest in knowing about the ethnic group grows and an awareness of discrimination increases; and achieved, when the role of ethnic group membership becomes more clear, and a secure sense of self as a member of the ethnic group develops (Phinney, 1996).

While Phinney's (1992) model outlines three developmental phases, her measure originally led to one score for ethnic identity achievement made up of scores from two subscales, Achievement (encompassing both exploration and resolution) and Ethnic Behaviors and Practices, though the latter consisted of only two items. Interestingly, Phinney's (1992) model did not combine "affirmation" with achievement, and she proposed that either positive or negative affect toward your group could be associated with the resolution of your ethnic identity. However, her measure, the Multigroup Ethnic Identity Measure (MEIM), employed items that did combine the two concepts under "achievement" (Cokley, 2007; Umaña-Taylor, et al., 2004). A revised version of Phinney's measure (MEIM-R; Phinney & Ong, 2007) now conceptualizes ethnic identity development as consisting of two distinct factors or scales: exploration and commitment, though the latter still combines the affirmation and achievement concepts.

The Ethnic Identity Scale (EIS; Umaña-Taylor et al., 2004) assesses the three components of the ethnic identity development process—exploration, resolution, and affirmation—as distinct subscales. It does not assess ethnic practices and behaviors, which are often assessed by acculturation measures (Cuéllar, Arnold, & Maldonado,1995), a concept to be discussed later in this chapter. Ethnic identity models specific to Latinos have also been developed (Bernal, Knight, Ocampo, Garza, & Cota, 1993; Ruiz, 1990) and typically include the developmental tasks presented above. We have taken the time to introduce you to some of the theoretical and measurement issues so that you will be better informed about the complexities of conceptualizing and assessing this ethnic identity development, and have a deeper understanding of the factors that make up the process. For the purposes of introducing you to this process, we will use Phinney's framework as a guide, while noting the important distinction between the achievement/resolution process and feelings of affirmation and belonging.

A Personal Journey into Ethnic Identity and Ethnic Self-Identification

While not formally a part of the ethnic identity development process outlined above, changes in ethnic self-identification may be a byproduct or result of this process. As people go through the stages of ethnic identity development, they will choose an ethnic self-label that reflects how they are experiencing their ethnic group memberships at that point in time. Our stories of ethnic identity development shared below are mainly organized according to changes in self-identification, but note other factors involved in the process which were mentioned earlier: exploration, resolution/achievement, and affirmation.

As noted above, during the initial stage of ethnic identity, "there is little interest in or concern for ethnicity" (Phinney 1995; p. 60). Its development occurs as part of the basic sense of self that develops in the early years of life. It is, in that sense, a "core" part of the personality, and it happens in the same way that all socialization happens. It is inculcated in us by our way of life; it is subtle, and occurs under the radar. We do not have to be told, "You are Mexicano (or Colombiano, Cubano, Dominicano, etc.)." We simply are because we live it.

Nicolás

Mexicano...

When I was a child, I lived in San Juan, a small town located in the center of the Rio Grande Valley of Texas. My parents, grandparents, siblings, maternal and paternal aunts, uncles, and cousins also lived there. We were all Mexicanos. We all spoke Spanish; we listened to Spanish radio, and when we went to the drive-in cinema we watched Spanish-speaking Mexicano movie stars. Everyone who played an important role in my life was a Mexicano, and I was a Mexicano. I never questioned that, and I was ignorant of the fact that I might be, or might call myself, something different.

Michele

Hispanic...

When I was young, I attended a predominately White European American elementary school, which reflected the composition of the neighborhood in which I lived. To my knowledge, there were only two other Hispanic families in the neighborhood. I'm sure this wasn't entirely true, but those two families had children in my grade level, so I was aware of them. I thought the only Hispanics in the world were my immediate family, these other two families, and my relatives. I knew that we were different because of our last name, my black hair, some of the food we ate, my grandparents who only spoke English, and our relatives in the Rio Grande Valley. In spite of these cultural connections, we only spoke English in my home; it was my first language, and our lifestyle was very mainstream. I guess I figured that all Hispanics were the kind of Hispanics we were.

We acquire some awareness that there are ethnic differences among people because we begin to experience ethnic labeling at a young age. "Are you Mexican?" is a question commonly heard in elementary schools in Texas and the Southwest, as others try to understand exactly who we were, even if we ourselves (as children) do not yet have a clear sense of our ethnicity. Presumably, a similar question is asked in other parts of the country: "Are you Cuban?" in Florida, or "Are you Puerto Rican?" in New York. When and to what extent we become aware of our ethnicity depends on our surroundings. In an environment in which everyone is similar to us, we may not give our own, or anyone else's, ethnic identity much thought. However, if we are raised in an ethnically or culturally diverse environment, we may have a different experience; or if we relocate to a more diverse environment, we may start to give our ethnic group membership more thought. This process may also occur in reverse. If you learn about your ethnicity as a "minority" in an environment that is predominately non-Latino, then a move to an area that is more heavily populated by Latinos can also serve as an encounter experience, where previously formed ideas about your ethnic group membership begin to be challenged.

Regardless of the environment in which one is raised, adolescents have a better sense of the issue than elementary school children, who are somewhat tentative in their attributions of ethnic identity. Their comments about ethnicity tend to be more definitive. In middle and high school, comments like "She's Mexican" or "He's Cuban" may be heard as ethnic labels attributed to one another. Conversely, statements such as "You're not really Mexican" and "coconut" (brown on the outside and white on the inside) are also heard, as in-group members try to define who belongs and who does not. Finally, it is during adolescence that most of us first choose a term for our ethnic self-identification, rather than using a term that has been chosen for us.

Nicolás

Mexican American...

When I entered elementary school, sometimes I was told that I was Latin American and other times that I was Spanish American. It made no sense to me, because for me, Mexicano translated into "Mexican," not Latin American or Spanish American. As I studied and learned about history, and experienced life in general, I figured that I had to fit in somewhere. The idea that I was American of Mexican descent made perfect sense to me. My grandparents were born in Mexico, my parents and I were born in the United States: I must be *Mexican American.*

Michele

Mexican American or American Mexican?

Upon entering the sixth grade, desegregation was enacted in our city. I was bussed across town from a predominately White middle-class area to a school in a lower socioeconomic status, predominately Latino, neighborhood. My first shock came at realizing that there were more of "us" than I had realized. Like I mentioned before, in my little world, few Hispanics existed outside of my family. However, I soon became aware that the students of Mexican descent from the "Eastside" did not consider me to be one of them. The "us" I thought I was a part of quickly crumbled. I felt rejected and confused. I was resented for the advantages I had; the advantages my parents had worked so hard to get for me. I knew I wasn't White, but now I wasn't Mexican enough, either. I had come to think of myself as Mexican American, but I felt more "American Mexican" in my new environment.

We become aware of ethnicity in the process of coming in contact with people of different backgrounds, and in doing so we gain awareness about ethnic differences and reflect on our own ethnic identity. We might try to make sense of ethnicity by asking direct questions, reading, or simply by observing those around us (exploration). In any case, the process is part of normal development, and by the time we reach late adolescence, we have a relatively clear preference for our ethnic self-identification and a developing sense of our ethnic identity. If we are asked, "Are you Mexican (Cuban, Puerto Rican, etc.)?" we can readily answer the question, by affirmation ("Yes") or clarification ("No, I'm Costa Rican"). Coming to terms with and establishing our ethnic identity (resolution) may be a relatively smooth and seamless process for many, part-and-parcel of the larger adolescent task of identity development. However, for others this process may be complicated, especially when we suddenly find ourselves in an environment that is culturally different from the one in which we were raised.

Nicolás

Culture Shock...

We moved to Austin, Texas in 1971, my senior year in high school. I entered Travis High School the first day of my senior year, and was pleased to see so many brown faces around me. I will never forget, however, the first name that was read off by the teacher that day, "Aglar," to which an obviously Mexican American student answered "here." I thought, "He looks Mexican American, but he must be Anglo." I later discovered that his name was "Aguilar," that none of my peers spoke Spanish, and that I spoke better Spanish than the Spanish teacher. There was nothing in Austin that was Mexicano, Mexican, or even Mexican American, as I conceived it to be.

Nothing in my simple, rural, "culturally sheltered" life in the Rio Grande Valley of Texas could have prepared me for what I encountered in Austin. I later learned that my experience was called "culture-shock." In my ignorance, I blamed my peers for their lack of Spanish language skills and unfamiliarity with things "Mexican" (as I knew them). I assumed that they did not speak Spanish because they did not wish to do so, and I assumed that they purposely chose not to be Mexicano or even Mexican American. I rejected them, as I thought they had rejected our culture.

The experience of culture shock can turn your whole world upside down. Things that seem perfectly clear no longer make any sense. The experience can be quite traumatic, and for some it can have a serious negative psychological impact on your life; see, for example, *Down These Mean Streets* (Thomas, 1967) and *Hunger of Memory* (Rodriguez, 1982).

According to Phinney, the second stage of ethnic identity development is a process of exploration, "an effort to learn more about one's ethnicity and its meaning" (1995, p. 60). Many of us become interested in learning about our culture at some point in our lives, and ethnicity becomes a very important part of our overall identity. This edifying process counteracts culture shock and culminates in a sense of grounding and belonging. This is the third stage of ethnic identity development, where there is a commitment to one's ethnic group and an examined understanding of that group membership. See *When I was Puerto Rican* (Santiago, 1993) and *Burro Genius* (Villaseñor, 2004) for personal stories about arriving at an achieved ethnic identity.

Nicolás

Chicano...

During my teens in the 1960s, I was superficially aware of the struggle between my people and the established order. In connection with that I heard the term "Chicano," and I called myself a Chicano, even though I had no clear sense of what it meant or of all that it symbolized. As I entered young adulthood, I began to study Mexican American history. I learned about Mexican Americans, Chicanos, Mexicanos, Tejanos, *Californios,* La Raza, Mexico, the Aztecs, and Aztlán. The more I learned about my people and culture, the more I liked the term "Chicano." I came to find that the term fit emotionally, intellectually, and politically.

More importantly, I became aware of my mistake; my peers in Austin had not given up our language and our culture; they were living it, just differently from the way I had experienced it. Being in the "minority," they had experienced more severe oppression than I had. Accepting this, I was able to reconnect with my people in Austin.

Michele

Reclaiming my roots...

By the time I reached college, I had a sense that having been raised "American Mexican" by my parents was a direct result of the discrimination they had faced as children (such as getting their hands hit with rulers for speaking Spanish in school) and their wish that we have a better life than they did. I also realized that I wanted back the part of my culture that this process of internalized discrimination had taken from my generation. I took Spanish classes to improve the "Espanglish" I had learned from my grandparents, joined the Latino student group on campus, and through mixing with other Latinos who had gained access to the private liberal arts college I was attending, started learning about the social justice issues that impacted Latinos. By the time I reached graduate school, I had made a firm commitment to "give back"; to use my educated status to help other Latinos. I studied Spanish in Mexico, participated in and initiated practica where I could conduct therapy with Latinos, and studied family therapy in Spain for two months. During my internship, 80% of my clients were Latino; much of the therapy I conducted was in Spanish; and suddenly I was the "expert" on serving the same to lower-SES, less privileged, and predominately Spanish-monolingual Mexican community that I felt had rejected me so many years before.

It is important to note that even though one has reached the final stage in Phinney's model—having an examined, achieved, or resolved ethnic identity—sociological, political, or personal factors can cause one to re-examine and/or reformulate that identity. In essence, one can revert back to a process of exploration and reflection before once more reaching a point of resolution. Additionally, while our own processes resulted in a positive sense of belonging or affirmation to our ethnic groups, other people's journeys may lead them to conclude that their particular Latino ethnic group membership is not salient or relevant at that point in their lives. As mentioned earlier, this identity development process might happen several times in a lifespan.

Nicolás

Mexicano to Latino

It took several years of study, exploration, examination, and maturation for me to reach a sense of commitment or achieved ethnic identity. That identity, however, did not last forever. It was not destabilized to the extent that it was by the culture-shock experience, but sociopolitical changes have caused me to re-examine my ethnic group identification. That adjustment to my ethnic identity is attributed to the changes in immigration patterns that have occurred over the last two decades, which resulted in an influx of people from Central and South America into the U.S. This sociopolitical factor has caused me to reflect on how I might be a part of or fit into that group of people, and today I have a different sense of my ethnic identity than I did twenty years ago. Today, I am Latino.

Michele

Mexican American, Latina, Chicana

I have reached a point in my life where I know what being Mexican American means for me, and I am comfortable with that. I know that there are those for whom it means something different. I no longer worry about "not being Mexican enough." I know my Mexican heritage and how it has influenced my life. I also recognize the privilege that I have, not only because of being educated but also because I am a light-skinned, highly acculturated, yet still bicultural, Latina. I prefer to self-identify as Mexican American, but don't mind being referred to as Latina, because I recognize the history, culture, and oppression that ties me to other Latinos. I also don't mind being referred to as Chicana. While it was a movement before my time, my grandparents and my parents (when they were younger) were migrant workers, so I value and respect those who fought for the rights and safety of farm workers. Even with this fairly settled sense of who I am ethnically, I find myself searching for more connections. Having lost all of my grandparents and now my mother, I have an even stronger desire to learn, preserve, and reconnect with my Mexican roots, and to pass them on to my children, and so the exploration continues.

Ethnic Identity Models Applied to Latino Clients

While you may have found our personal ethnic identity development stories of interest, as a counselor in training eager to assist your Latino clients you may be wondering how the concept of ethnic identity development will be helpful to you. In other words, how does a theory about ethnic identity translate into competently counseling Latinos? Being aware that ethnic identity is a unique process for each Latino individual, will better prepare you to assist your clients. Without a working understanding of this socialization process, you might think that someone who is Puerto Rican, Cuban, and so on has a similar experience with regard to ethnicity as every other person in that ethnic group. As is evidenced by our stories, this is not the case.

It is unlikely that a client will ever come to a first session reporting that she or he is "experiencing issues surrounding ethnic identity development." In fact, most laypeople are not familiar with the concept. However, if we look at the stages proposed by Phinney, we can see that it is possible that clients may speak about being out of touch with their backgrounds, disinterested in their ethnicity, or even resentful that they belong to their ethnic group. All of these may be viewed as expressions of the unexamined stage. Or, you may have clients who express wanting to know more about their ethnic backgrounds, or who feel they are being discriminated against or are starting to see discrimination operating in the world around them. Often, people in this exploration phase have had some type of encounter experience. Such an experience is one in which a person is awakened to the saliency of his or her ethnic group membership. As mentioned before, for some it is a change of environment, often one where the ethnic demographics are considerably different; for others, it is entering a relationship with an ethnically different other, or taking an ethnic studies course. Finally, individuals in the examined stage may express very clear ideas of what their ethnic background means to them on a day-to-day basis and in their current relationships. However, this does not mean that these clients will not experience conflict around their ethnicity, only that such conflict may not center around discovering the meaning of one's ethnicity. It may instead involve negotiating a resolved ethnic identity with other identities, or with others who do not hold similar beliefs about their ethnic backgrounds.

The elements of the ethnic identity stages as described above will most likely not appear in isolation, but will be intertwined with other emotional and behavioral concerns. An example may help to illustrate the process. Suppose your Puerto Rican client, Marc, reports that he grew up in a predominantly White European American neighborhood, but now finds himself working with other Puerto Ricans who appear to have more ties to the Island and their ethnic culture. He reports feeling uncomfortable, like he does not "fit in." Marc is probably not going to come out and say, "I'm having an ethnic identity crisis." In fact, he may identify the issue more as a work environment concern than an ethnic identity development challenge. Marc may talk about his own socialization experience with regard to ethnicity, and he may talk about not really feeling attached to the culture, and feeling unsure if he wants to be more attached. On the one hand, he was comfortable with the label "Puerto Rican" as he has experienced it, but now he wonders if, in comparison to his coworkers, he is "really Puerto Rican enough." This would be a case where you could guide him through discussion and exploration of the various aspects of the ethnic identity process, and also assess to what extent he has previously explored his culture and his ethnic group membership. You might query him about other significant "contact" (encounter) experiences that made him question this aspect of his identity. Finally, you would help to summarize and clarify the information he has presented, and in doing so facilitate his own unique achieved or resolved sense of ethnic identity. Throughout this process it would be beneficial to use your empathy skills, along with other basic counseling techniques, to validate the challenging feelings that Marc may experience as part of this exploration and discussion.

Note that an examined or resolved sense of identity does not always mean that someone will choose to be strongly identified with his or her ethnic background, nor does it mean that this identity will rank highly for that person among other identities such as gender, religion, or sexual orientation. An examined identity is exactly as the term indicates: that the person has explored the issue and has not foreclosed on the process of figuring out his or her unique and personal meaning of ethnicity. As mentioned earlier, some scholars, like Umaña-Taylor et al. (2004) conceptualized "affirmation" as a separate part of ethnic identity from resolution, specifically because the outcome of the exploration and achievement process may be laden with positive or negative feelings toward one's ethnic group. Phinney (1990) found that individuals with an examined ethnic identity tend to have higher self-esteem. To review, assisting a client with ethnic identity issues would likely entail the following steps:

1. Being familiar with the concept of ethnic identity development.
2. Educating clients about this developmental process, including normalizing feelings and experiences they may encounter in each phase.
3. Supporting clients as they experience a variety of feelings, which may include resentment, anger, excitement, and sadness as they wrestle with each stage of the process.
4. Facilitating the exploration process by suggesting ways that clients may explore their ethnic group traditions and history, such as talking to family members—especially older ones—about their experiences, taking ethnic studies courses, traveling to the country of their oldest remembered ancestors, and attending cultural events.
5. Encouraging clients to stay engaged in the process even when others around them may not be supportive or may not like the expression of the stages that they are experiencing.
6. Supporting whatever conclusion clients come to about their ethnic group membership.

RACIAL IDENTITY

Now that we have spent some time discussing ethnic identity development, we turn to examining racial identity development among Latinos, a topic that for this group is seldom discussed and has taken a back seat to examinations of ethnicity and ethnic identity. To be clear, when we refer to racial identity development, we are discussing a process by which people come to understand their racial group membership and how they make sense of racism. This differs from the ethnic identity development process discussed previously. Ethnicity deals with connections to one's oldest remembered ancestors by way of language, customs, foods, dress, and so on. Race, on the other hand, deals with the socially constructed categorization system we use in the U.S., which is based on skin color and phenotype (hair texture, facial features). Racial categorization is a system that was originally organized to advantage some and disadvantage others, and continues to do so to this day.

Much discussion concerning racial identity has taken place within the field of Counseling Psychology (Carter, 1997; Cokley, 2007; Cross, 1995; Cross & Vandiver, 2001; Helms, 1995). However, racial identity has generally remained a Black and White issue, leaving a paucity of research regarding this construct as it applies to Latinos. The conceptualization of race itself is problematic in this population, and some would argue that this is true in general. Latinos are usually thought of as one ethnic group, when in reality we represent numerous groups, and terms such as "Latino" and "Hispanic" are pan-ethnic labels. Sometimes Latinos are discussed alongside Asian Americans, Whites, and so on as if we represent a single racial group. As discussed earlier, Latinos are by definition biracial or multiracial, being comprised of Black, White, and Indigenous backgrounds (Santiago-Rivera, Arredondo, & Gallardo-Cooper, 2002).

The United States Census has conceptualized Latinos in many ways. From 1940 to 1970, race was decided by the census taker. Interestingly, before self-reporting of race, 93.3% of Hispanics were classified as White. After people began categorizing themselves in 1980, only 57.7 % of Hispanics classified themselves as White (Rodriguez, 2000). While there seems to be some recognition by Latinos that they are not just White, there remains much confusion. When the 2000 census included for the first time the option of selecting "Some Other Race" in addition to the five standard categories (White, Black or African-American, Asian, American Indian and Alaskan Native, and Native Hawaiian and Other Pacific Islander), some 42% of Hispanics selected this new category and another 6% marked two or more racial categories. Latinos were virtually alone in moving away from the standard racial categories. In the 2000 census, Latinos made up 97% of the respondents picking the "Some Other Race" category (Pew Hispanic Center & Kaiser Family Foundation, 2002). It will be interesting to track the development of how Latinos categorize themselves racially in the future. While the 2010 census numbers are not available as of this writing, data from the 2008 American Community Survey indicate that the number of Latinos classifying themselves as "Some Other Race" dropped to 30.4%, with 62.5% choosing "White" as their racial classification; a notable shift from the 2000 census figures noted above.

Some racial identity models such as the Racial/Cultural Identity Development Model (R/CID; Sue and Sue, 2003) have been applied to Latinos, but they often appear to be referring to ethnicity, not race, or they mix the two concepts together. Furthermore, they usually treat Latinos as a racially homogeneous group, when in actuality some Latinos would be socially perceived as Black, while many Latinos have light skin and can "pass" as White in some circumstances. Even models of biracial identity development (Kerwin and Ponterotto, 1995) seem to focus more on choice of affiliation with one racial group or another, or acceptance of one's "differentness," as opposed to dealing with issues of privilege and racism. Furthermore, these biracial identity models seem to be addressing the offspring of mixed racial couples, thereby representing a "recent" biracial generation. Latinos have been bi- or multiracial for hundreds of years, so these models may be inappropriate for this population. Here, we use Helms' (1995) White and People of Color Racial Identity Ego Statuses Models as a reference point for this discussion, because these models refer specifically to the manner in which people interpret racial information.

Helms' Racial Identity Ego Statuses and Information-Processing Models

The People of Color Model, based on Helms' (1995) original Black racial identity model, consists of five statuses: Conformity, Dissonance, Immersion/Emersion, Internalization, and Integrative Awareness. Individuals in the Conformity status are characterized by the rejection of their own racial group and have preferences for the dominant racial group (White Americans). Ambivalence or conflict about racial and cultural attitudes toward one's own racial group and the White group characterize the status of Dissonance. In the Immersion/Emersion status, individuals immerse themselves in and idealize their own race and culture while rejecting and holding negative attitudes about White individuals. Internalization occurs when individuals have a positive attitude toward their own racial group, use internal criteria for racial self-definition, and have the capacity to assess and respond to members of the dominant racial group objectively. Integrative Awareness is the status in which individuals value their own group identity as well as recognizing similarities between themselves and members of other oppressed groups.

Helms' model of White racial identity development consists of six stages: Contact, Disintegration, Reintegration, Pseudoindependence, Immersion/Emersion, and Autonomy. According to Helms (1995), White individuals may begin at a point where they are oblivious to racism and their participation in it (Contact); they may also not think of themselves as being "White"; instead they just experience themselves as "normal." When faced with a situation or information in which racism is present, they may no longer be able to deny their racial group membership and its accompanying advantage, and Disintegration begins to occur. Helms further proposes that this status may be too painful and that some individuals may experience Reintegration where there is intolerance for other racial groups and idealization of one's own. After possibly moving through a Pseudoindependence status, where there is a superficial commitment to tolerating other groups and understanding racism, individuals become immersed in a search for a deep and personal understanding of racism and one's role in it (Immersion/Emersion). Finally, the person reaches Autonomy, where there is a realistic appraisal of one's racial group, one not based on false notions of supremacy, and the person commits to relinquish privilege to the extent possible and to actively oppose racism at all levels.

Although Helms' model was originally cast in terms of developmental stages, Helms (1995) has since suggested that individuals should not necessarily be classified as having one particular racial identity status; rather, they have schemas (ways of thinking) of varying relevance to multiple racial identity statuses. Thus, an individual may exhibit characteristics of more than one racial identity status, and these may vary in degree and frequency. When the Helms model was used to explore racial identity development in Asian Americans, for whom this concept is complicated and understudied—much as it is in Latinos—cluster analysis revealed "profiles" in which more than one "status" appeared to capture the participants' thinking about race and racial group membership (Chen, LePhuoc, Guzmán, Rude, & Dodd, 2006). Additionally, it should be understood that these models represent theory which is still being tested through research. The racial identity process may not look like this for all individuals, and not all individuals may experience each of these statuses, or experience them in the order presented.

As was highlighted in our discussion of ethnic identity development, it should be noted that the translation of Helms' model of racial identity into a measure of racial identity, the Racial Identity Attitude Scale (RIAS; Parham & Helms, 1981), has not been without its challenges. Concerns have been raised about the psychometric properties of the RIAS (Cokley, 2007). We encourage you to look at other conceptualizations and models of racial identity development, such as the Cross Racial Identity Scale (CRIS; Vandiver, Fhagen-Smith, Cokley, Cross Jr., & Worrell, 2001), to further inform your thinking about this concept.

Using Racial Identity Models to Assist Latino Clients

As was mentioned with regard to ethnic identity, it is unlikely that clients will come in asking for counseling around racial identity development issues. However, clients may speak of discrimination experiences. Some of these experiences may be linked more to ethnic discrimination; ridicule and prejudice due to ethnic group membership, food preferences, dress, or language (either lack of knowledge of English or a notable accent). Racism surrounds prejudice concerning skin color, phenotype (often facial features which are more Indigenous) or racial group attributes in general (in the case of Latinos, appearing to be something other than White). While both ethnic prejudice and racism may be experienced by Latinos, and both are unjust and painful, counselors should understand the subtle differences.

Often, Latinos are relatively unaware of their racial group membership. They tend to identify ethnically, and often when asked what race they are, they will answer "Hispanic" or "Latino," not recognizing their multiracial identities. Racial group membership is important because Latinos, while they may not consciously view race as important for them, can see salient race issues playing out in their lives. Take, for instance, Latina girls and women who feel they must straighten their hair, preferring silky straight to naturally curly in order to be seen as beautiful by the standards of U.S. society. Furthermore, comments in the Latino community regarding skin color are abundant. Parents and relatives often rejoice when a light-skinned baby is born, or children are admonished for being out in the sun too long lest they get "too dark." In the film *Skin Deep* (Reid & Wood, 1995), Judy, a college student of Mexican descent, shares a story that her uncle told her and her sister: "You're dark but you're still pretty." As a whole, Latinos have been indoctrinated to celebrate their European features and downplay or dislike their Indigenous qualities. Latinos who are very dark-skinned or have very curly hair due to having Black ancestors have a particularly difficult time, as they may be categorized as "Black" and experience the racism felt by African Americans while their Latino group membership may not be recognized.

Light-skinned Latino clients may achieve success by being able to "pass" in many situations, but then may share stories of being ostracized by other Latinos. They may be called White or "sell-out." Because Latinos have such a variety of European roots mixed in with their Indigenous roots, some may be very fair-skinned and have light-colored eyes. Latinos who have one parent who is White European American may also face rejection from Latino peers. While light-skinned Latinos are likely still not accepted fully as "White" and may themselves still experience discrimination from Whites, it is still important for them to recognize and claim the privilege they have based on lighter skin, light eyes, or straight hair. As mentioned time and time again, we are part Spanish, part European, and therefore part White. To the extent this is visible, Latinos must explore the aspects of the White racial identity process that applies to them.

The steps to supporting racial identity development in Latinos are similar to those of ethnic identity development: normalize feelings, encourage exploration, and support personal and unique conclusions. More specifically, reflecting the tasks outlined by Helms (1995), a counselor might:

1. Assess to what extent the client is aware of racial group membership and issues surrounding racism.
2. Evaluate how and to what degree racial identity issues may be affecting the client and his or her presenting problem. A counselor should not force the exploration of racial identity issues where there does not seem to be a relevance or readiness, but not being ready and willing to discuss these issues may lead the client to think that this topic is off-limits or unsafe to discuss.
3. Inform the client of the racial identity development process. You do not have to use technical terms, naming each status; instead simply share with the client the challenges, ideas, and tasks surrounding the statuses.
4. Validate the painful feelings that often accompany the exploration of issues of race and racism.
5. Support clients in drawing their own conclusions about the meaning of their racial group membership and the role they would like to take, if any, in dealing with racism.
6. Facilitate clients' exploration of the areas in which they have choice and power in dealing with racism. For dark-skinned Latinos, this may mean exploring areas where they can fight racism, and other areas where they may need to learn how to cope with it. For light-skinned Latinos, this may mean balancing an exploration of both discrimination and privilege.

Where advantage does exist, there may be an examination of how they can use their privilege to assist other Latinos and people of color and use their status with Whites to make change.

WORLDVIEW

We all have ways of making sense of the world, our lives, and the events around us. This conceptual framework is sometimes referred to in the multicultural literature as "worldview." A conceptualization of worldview encompasses such elements as time focus, social relations, view of human activity, and relationships to nature (Sue & Sue, 2003). You may have heard discussion of the "Eurocentric" worldview, or the philosophy of life that is held by mainstream White European American culture. Such a view includes the concept of rugged individualism, a future time orientation, a focus on the nuclear family, and a "pull yourself up by your bootstraps" mentality about work and success. These may or may not be views that you subscribe to, but it is important to recognize that many Latino clients either do not subscribe to such views or do so to a lesser extent that non-Latinos. In the following pages, we will examine some of the cultural scripts or values that may influence the worldview of Latino individuals.

CULTURAL SCRIPTS

A Latino worldview consists, among other things, of a more present-focused time orientation, warmth in personal relationships, a focus on collective well-being versus individualism, and a trust in fate or a higher power to take care of concerns and problems. Cultural scripts, which can also be thought of as cultural values, make up and influence the worldview of Latinos. These cultural scripts may provide us with information on how Latinos experience, interpret, and react to many social situations and problems. They also guide the gender roles that Latinos play out in their relationships and the manner in which they seek help and healing. Díaz-Guerrero (1967) conceptualized cultural scripts as "sociocultural premises," conscious or unconscious culturally significant assumptions upon which a given group bases its thinking, feeling, and behavior. It is important to remember that not all Latinos subscribe equally to the ideas we will discuss here. Level of acculturation, ethnic identity, education, and generation all impact the extent to which a person's life reflects these values. Assessing the extent to which a client subscribes to these values will be discussed at the end of the chapter after some of the cultural scripts have been presented.

Throughout this section, and when we discuss the concept of acculturation later in this chapter, we often use the word "traditional." In the literature, traditional has often been equated with values reflective of recent immigrants or those in the U.S. who are closer to the experience of their native country. However, this thinking may be too simplistic. For example, we cannot assume that a recent immigrant from Mexico or a second-generation Mexican American will hold more traditional values than a third-generation Mexican American across any number of issues related to worldview. Societal practices, laws, politics, and customs are not static in Mexico, or any other country outside the U.S. They are constantly changing, as they are here. For example, while we may be inclined to think of traditional Latino values as being more conservative around the issue of same-sex relationships, same-sex civil unions and marriages are performed in Mexico City and the Mexican supreme court has ruled that they must be honored throughout the country (Allende, 2010). Most large cities in the U.S. do not allow for either civil unions or gay marriages, other states do not recognize gay marriages allowed in a small number of states, and a hotly contested debate continues around the issue of gay marriage nationwide. Therefore, when we say "traditional," we mean on a continuum from more conservative to more progressive with respect to ideas or values, without implying that the native country is situated at the former and the U.S. at the latter.

Personalismo

Latino clients may appreciate a greater degree of personal warmth in counseling relationships than their European American counterparts. This may mean taking more time for small-talk before getting down to business, or initiating a handshake in a field which has taught us to be hypervigilant about touching our clients in any way. Something as simple as asking a Latino client how his or her family is before beginning a session will convey a sense of caring for the client as a person, and not simply as a client or patient. It also demonstrates an appreciation for the family, *la familia*, as an important part of Latino culture. A therapist may also want to use self-disclosure to establish rapport and a greater climate of warmth and trust with Latino clients. As with all clients, clinical judgment and the therapist's personal comfort level should guide self-disclosure. You should not feel obligated to answer inappropriate or highly personal questions for the sake of making a client more comfortable.

Understanding the value of *personalismo* is important for both the beginning or seasoned therapist as it relates to accepting gifts from clients. Part of this cultural value involves showing appreciation to others and being interpersonally sensitive. Along these lines, refusing to accept a gift from a Latino client could be considered very rude and hurtful by the client. Oftentimes our decisions, such as thinking we cannot accept gifts from clients, are based on ethical codes that only reflect the values of mainstream European Americans (Sue & Sue, 2003). Just as many of our theoretical orientations were shaped without the perspectives of people of color, so were our ethical codes and standards of clinical conduct. Again, we tell students that if a client wants to give you an inappropriate gift (like a diamond ring or cash), however tempting, you should not accept it. However, clients often simply want to give a *regalo* (gift) they purchased in their country of origin, or a traditional food such as tamales, as a way of thanking the therapist for his or her help. As with any client, it is important to discuss with the client what the gift means or symbolizes, and to do the same for the meaning of the gift to the therapist. This will avoid any misunderstanding or confusion around expectations that the gift may create. In this way, it is possible to combine traditional clinical judgment with the cultural framework being proposed here.

Finally, it is recommended that therapists pay special attention to power dynamics with clients. As discussed in detail in Chapter 2, Latinos have been the victims of discrimination in the U.S. for many years. While it is impossible to escape the "one-down" power position of clients in therapeutic relationships, an egalitarian approach with an emphasis on personalismo may help create a climate in which a Latino client can feel safe and comfortable. However, it should be noted that many Latinos expect a hierarchical relationship to exist with professionals, so while the therapist should strive for warmth in the relationship, this should not be interpreted as adopting a loose, informal, or "laid back" approach.

Familismo

Latinos place a great amount of importance on the family, both nuclear and extended. This focus on the family is characterized by a strong sense of obligation to take care of family members, even to the point of sacrificing one's own needs or desires. There is also a strong sense of interdependence, loyalty, and attachment among members of the family (Cuéllar, Arnold, and González, 1995).

Michele

The importance of family...

I sometimes reflect upon the fact that even though I am well into adulthood, with a family of my own, I still see or talk to at least half of my six siblings on a daily basis. For my children, aunts and uncles are a daily part of their lives, not just people they see twice a year on holidays and school vacations. For the two years that my mother was terminally ill with breast cancer, my work never came before her healthcare needs, and there was no question that she would move in with me during the final months of her illness. I remember people asking me if we would take her to a hospital, nursing home, or some other inpatient hospice care for her final weeks. I emphatically replied that no, we would not. It was me, my uncle, my brothers and sisters (and yes, some hired help), who transferred her to her wheelchair, moved her to the bedside toilet, and later, when she lost control of all of her bodily functions, turned her, changed her, and fed her. She died in my home, and there was no question that it would happen any differently, even though I also had a 1-year-old infant to care for during the last stage of her illness and her passing. That's what *familismo* means: to put your family before yourself, even if it costs you.

Unfortunately, the demands of education and careers in the U.S. do not conform to the expectations of the cultural script of familismo. Latinos and Latinas find themselves caught between wanting to get ahead in life, often for the eventual benefit of the family, and needing to tend to their family obligations. It can be a hard choice for a young Latino to go away to school or move to another town for that great job. Even when success is achieved, the requirements of high-level positions are often at odds with putting your family first. This can cause a great deal of stress and may contribute to why Latinos often may not rise to the highest positions in their fields. Unfortunately, in the past, the psychological professions have mistakenly characterized these close relationships and ties among Latinos as enmeshment. As with other concepts we will mention in this chapter, it is important to look at outcomes. If Latino clients are not happy with their roles in their families, or the manner in which their families function, then this is certainly an area for exploration in therapy. The role of the counselor here is one of facilitator, helping Latinos to retain the strength of the cultural script of familismo while allowing themselves to grasp the personal and individual dreams they may have for themselves.

Fatalismo

Another cultural script that may influence the worldview of Latinos is the concept of fatalism, or *fatalismo*, which refers most generally to the extent to which people feel their destinies are outside of their control, but also encompasses religious views, as well as a present-time orientation (Cuéllar et al., 1995). Empirical validations of this concept have found mixed results. Rotter's (1990) internal-external control theory refers to the degree to which persons expect that an outcome of their behavior is contingent on their own behavior versus chance, luck, fate, or the control of powerful others. However, through a factor analysis of Rotter's I-E scale (1966, as cited in Garza, 1977), Garza found that Mexican Americans may conceptualize fatalism differently from non-Latino Whites.

In line with Garza's (1977) findings, Sue and Sue (1990) caution that it is important to distinguish between various meanings of externality when dealing with culturally diverse clients, as these meanings may have to do with a belief in chance-luck, religious beliefs, or political forces (racism and discrimination). Falicov (1998) states that there are two theories of fatalism: a "deficit-oriented" theory where fatalism is seen as increasing psychological distress, and a "resource-oriented" theory where it may be used to selectively cope with losses that are beyond one's control, such as incurable disease or an unexpected death (p. 150; Neff & Hoppe, 1993). When working with Latino clients it is important that cultural scripts such as fatalism be viewed in an interactive sense, not a simplistic one. For instance, fatalism may be a disadvantage within the context of U.S. systems which require a future-oriented, planning focus, but a resource in other contexts, where releasing some control might be helpful. The former situation should be perceived more as a "cultural mismatch" than a deficit.

As a therapist, you are in a unique and important position to assist Latino clients in negotiating the process of integrating a fatalistic perspective with the mainstream U.S. worldview which generally emphasizes an internal locus of control. In determining whether the client's fatalistic view is harmful or helpful in any given situation, the therapist should carefully examine the outcome; that is, where is this perspective leading the client? For example, if a fatalistic attitude allows a terminally ill client to have a sense of peace that his or her life, and death, is "meant to be" or is in God's hands, then that may be a very calming and helpful attitude. However, this situation differs greatly from that of a cancer patient with some hope of recovery who refuses to seek treatment, because she believes that God will cure her if she is meant to be cured. In this case, you may want to explore with the client any fears or misconceptions about receiving treatment for her illness. You might also reassure the client that seeking treatment does not mean rejecting faith in God, and sharing a perspective such as "God helps those who help themselves" may allow for productive discussion.

However, it is also important to understand that a fatalistic viewpoint may stem from years of oppression. As discussed earlier, Latinos have received many messages that they are not in control of their own lives, from the hundreds of years that the Spaniards enslaved Indigenous people and Africans to more contemporary racism such as limiting their access to education and other opportunities in the twentieth century. Against this backdrop, it is easier to understand why a Latino adolescent may not believe that doing well in high school is going to make a difference in her future. It is hard to believe in the American dream when you have been repeatedly excluded from it. In this case, it is important for the therapist to acknowledge the context for why the client may feel that she does not have control, but to then examine the current evidence for this viewpoint. The therapist can help the client identify areas where she can make a difference and where she does have control, even if this is only centered around her attitude toward the situation. Then the therapist and client can work together to examine the most beneficial ways to cope with factors that are beyond her control.

TRADITIONAL GENDER ROLES

Machismo

Machismo is a Latino cultural script that, having been popularized by U.S. media, is often misconstrued by therapists; one reason for this is that the term (*macho*) from which *machismo* is derived has been integrated into U.S. vocabulary. The term "macho" is spelled and pronounced the same in English and Spanish, but it is defined differently in each language. In Spanish, the term simply means "male" or "masculine"; on the other hand, in English, it refers to a man who is aggressive, domineering, a womanizer, and unfaithful in marriage.

For the counselor interested in understanding Latino males, it is important to know that the concept of *macho* does play an important role in the socialization of Latino men, and that traditional Latino fathers often inculcate in their sons the idea of being macho, and therefore, being macho is a part of the Latino male self-concept. However, the concept of being macho, in the Latino sense, is an honorable one, and it includes pride, dignity, benevolence, courage, devotion, hard-work, sacrifice, responsibility, as well as other very positive qualities. In Spanish, we have a saying: *"Se cree muy macho"*, which means "He thinks he is very manly". This saying reflects the notion that some men portray a false sense of manhood; these men are not macho, they are *machista,* which conceptually is equivalent to a chauvinist Counselors need to be careful not to confuse and misuse the terms macho, as conceptualized in English, and macho as conceptualized in Spanish. The proper term used to describe men who are abusive is *machista.* It would be important to check with a Latino male client to see to what extent he subscribes to the macho versus machista self-concepts. In addition, counselors need to be aware of ways in which machista attitudes may affect the therapy process. At the outset, it may prevent Latino men from reaching out for help. There may be a sense that he should be able to solve his problems independently or that seeking help and sharing his emotions is a sign of weakness. In addition, a Latino whosubscribes to machista attitudes may prevent his family from getting services as well. If a Latino male does enter counseling, it will be very important to enforce the positive aspects of seeking help and reframe this as a strength, by talking about being macho and all positive attributes associated with this concept.

When working with a Latino family that is traditional in this respect, it would be important not to go over the father's head, so to speak. For instance, those of us who work with children may have been trained to try to engage the child first, perhaps focus on the child initially, to make him or her comfortable, but we would suggest that this approach may not be a good fit when working with a Latino family that is structured as we are discussing here. The counselor would not want to show a lack of respect for the head of the family, or the parental unit. Doing so may irreparably damage rapport.

If you do not subscribe to traditional gender roles, perhaps because you were not raised in a family that practiced them, or were raised in a family that did and are now reacting against them, you need to be aware of your own worldview on this issue. You need to watch your "countertransference"; in other words, your own "stuff" that you bring into the therapy room. Even if you disagree with a client's viewpoint, you need to be careful not to impose your own viewpoint on the client; this could be very damaging. Again, you need to examine to what extent the client's subscription to traditional gender roles is contributing to negative mental health outcomes, or is hindering the client from reaching goals that he or she would like to meet. Likewise, you should stay open to the idea that gender roles act as an asset for many Latinos. As mentioned before, factors such as education and acculturation may influence the extent to which Latinos and Latinas conform to traditional gender roles. We should never make assumptions, but must instead explore the client's perspective on such roles.

Marianismo

On the other side of the gender socialization issue is the role that is assigned to women in Latino culture, a cultural script referred to as *marianismo.* Above all else, sacrifice for the sake of the family and motherhood are respected. Women are expected to honor the model of the Virgin Mary; to be pure, nurturing, and to endure much suffering (Lopez-Baez, 1999). While the concept of marianismo does paint a picture of women as humble, it also suggests that they are spiritually stronger than men (Santiago-Rivera, Arredondo, & Gallardo-Cooper, 2002). The manner in which this cultural role may impact the therapeutic process is multifaceted. First of all, if a Latina is satisfied with a more traditional gender role, the therapist must take care to not try to "liberate" her encouraging her to subscribe to a more contemporary point of view. If such a woman is seeking change, it is important to consider the impact that changes to her perspective will have on her family system. It would be poor clinical practice to promote change in such a woman without assisting her in understanding the repercussions that such change will have for her partner and family.

It might be easy to think that many Latinas who are of later generations, are more acculturated, or who embrace less traditional gender roles due to exposure to education have simply "shed" the traditional expectations and formed a new idea of womanhood for themselves. Most of the time, this is far from the truth. A Latina who goes against traditional gender roles often faces challenges from family and society. If she wants to pursue post-secondary education, maybe even graduate or professional school, and then establish a career, this often means delaying marriage and motherhood. Such choices may bring disapproval from older generations. However, once established, Latinas who do wish to have a family may find themselves pressured from the workplace to make work a priority. Often, the value of putting family and motherhood first is still strong enough to make this situation extremely stressful. In *The Maria Paradox*, Gil and Vazquez (1996) discuss the dilemma faced by Latinas trying to negotiate traditional values and expectations with contemporary gender roles and the demands of the workplace. Latinas facing such role conflicts should be supported in negotiating the demands of family and career.

A discussion of gender roles would not be complete without giving attention to the way in which these issues intersect with sexual orientation for Latinos who identify as gay, lesbian, or bisexual. Racism and discrimination continue against people of color, but at least they are protected legally from discrimination. By contrast, in the U.S., it is often the laws themselves that discriminate against gay and lesbian individuals, preventing them from marrying, adopting children, and so forth. Imagine then the discrimination that Latinos and Latinas who are gay face as "double" minorities. In the case of Latinas, it is actually "triple": being a person of color, a woman, and a lesbian. Unfortunately, and perhaps most painfully, some of the worst discrimination comes from other Latinos, and often from their own families. Because being gay is often equated with being feminine, such a sexual orientation does not mesh well with a traditional machismo gender role. Being a lesbian almost certainly means that a woman will not become a "wife" and her chances of becoming a mother may diminish. For these reasons, being a lesbian may be seen as abandoning all that is important to the concept of marianismo. Therefore, gay, lesbian, and bisexual Latinos need an extraordinary amount of support and understanding from their counselors (Guarnero & Flaskerud, 2008). They have much to negotiate in the way of cultural gender role expectations. As when working with gay individuals from any ethnic or racial group, counselors need to explore their own views regarding sexual orientation, their heterosexual privilege if they are straight, and their "homoprejudices" (Barret, 1998), so that they may work compassionately and effectively with these clients.

TRADITIONS

There are a number of traditions in Latino culture which differ from those practiced or recognized by mainstream U.S. society. While there are too many to list here, giving a few examples may help to build some awareness of these different customs. In the U.S., we are familiar with adolescent girls celebrating their "Sweet Sixteen," but in Latino culture it is the fifteenth birthday that is special, and is celebrated with the *Quinceañera*, an observance that usually consists of attending a special mass and throwing a lavish party or dance. This type of celebration is probably practiced less frequently in later generations of Latinos in the U.S., but it has a significant history within the culture nonetheless.

An often misunderstood Latino (specifically Mexican) holiday is *Cinco de Mayo* (the fifth of May). In the U.S. this holiday is usually seen as an occasion to throw special happy hours and parties. It is also mistakenly thought of as "Mexican Independence Day," which is actually observed on September 16th. In reality, Cinco de Mayo is a remembrance of the victory over the French at the Battle of Puebla, Mexico in 1862. A final example of a special Latino holiday is *El Día de Los Reyes* (Three Kings Day). It takes place on January 6th, the day that, according to the biblical story, three wise men following a star and bearing gifts for baby Jesus arrived at his manger. In Latino countries, this day marks the climax of the holiday season, the day when children receive the most gifts ("Los Reyes Magos," 2005). This holiday is especially beloved and celebrated among Puerto Ricans.

A newer tradition that celebrates Latino culture in the U.S. is Hispanic Heritage Month, which occurs in September. The observance is positive in that it calls on people in the U.S. to focus on the contributions made by Latinos to this country, but it is also problematic. The fact that a month has to be "set aside" to honor Latino contributions to U.S. culture serves to highlight the fact that our educational system still does not teach, celebrate, and value on a daily basis the ways in which Latinos and Latino culture are inextricably intertwined with the history of this country and current U.S. society. As counselors in training, we need to recognize the strength and diversity of Latino culture, including its holidays, customs, and contributions to U.S. society. Sometimes counselors-in-training are afraid of showing ignorance about another culture, or they may be sensitive to the issue of people of color always having to explain themselves and teach others about their culture. While these are valid concerns, you can hardly go wrong by being genuinely interested in a person's culture, being honest about your ignorance, and sincerely seeking this information to develop a culturally sensitive approach to working with the person.

RELIGION AND SPIRITUALITY

Latinos are primarily Christian (93%), and within this religion 70% are Catholic (Espinosa, Elizondo, & Miranda, 2003). This stems from the history of the Spaniards bringing Catholicism to the New World as a tool for "civilizing" the Indigenous people. However, the native people and African slaves, being resilient as they were, found ways of incorporating their own spiritual concepts into Catholicism, which will be discussed later in this section. Latinos also participate in other major religions. Latinos who are Jewish may trace their origins to the Sephardic Jews who fled Spain in the fifteenth century during the Inquisition: other Latino Jews came to South America from Europe when Hitler came to power (Santiago-Rivera et al., 2002).

The large number of Latino Catholics counted in the U.S. is partly due to the large influx of Catholics from Latin America, especially Mexico, which has one of the highest rates of Catholicism in Latin America. The high percentage of Catholics is also attributable to the work of social programs that assist the poor, Catholic youth programs, and Catholic Charismatic movements (Espinosa et al., 2003). However, there is a significant demographic shift occurring among second and third generation Latinos. The Hispanic Churches in an American Public Life study found that the percentage of Latino Catholics drops from 74% among the first generation to 72% among the second, and 62% among the third generation. In conjunction with this, the percentage of Latino Protestants and "other Christians" increases from 15% among the first generation to 29% by the third generation (Espinosa et al., 2003). Therefore, it is important that counselors not assume that all Latino clients are Catholic. Most importantly, a therapist should find out what the client's experience of religion and spirituality is currently and has been in the past, and how this may be a resource in helping the client to heal.

Religious Beliefs and Practices

Latino Catholics observe a variety of religious traditions and ceremonies. Often, these practices are a blend of Indigenous influences and sometimes have their roots in African spiritual practices. *La Virgen de Guadalupe* (The Virgin of Guadalupe) is a special and much loved religious figure among Latinos of Mexican origin, as she is the patron saint of Mexico, and each year, thousands of Latinos make pilgrimages to the shrine of the Virgin in Mexico City. The Virgin appeared to Juan Diego in 1531, and imprinted her image on his *tilma*, or cloak. Scientific study has concluded that the image is truly miraculous (Johnston, 1981). For Cubans, Puerto Ricans, and Dominicans, other important religious figures include Christ and the Virgin Mary (often as Our Lady of Mercy). The practice of *Santeria* is a fusion of Catholicism and African traditions that is practiced by some Latinos, in which the African gods such as *Changó* and *Obatalá* are worshiped along with Our Lady of Mercy (Santiago-Rivera et al., 2002).

Religious beliefs are reflected in customs such as the building of altars in the home to show devotion to a saint or to remember loved ones. These altars may contain statues of favorite saints, candles, and pictures of deceased family members or friends. *El Día de los Muertos* (Day of the Dead) is a widely celebrated event among Mexicans and those of Mexican origin. Altars, as described above, are erected and adorned with food and other gifts. There are parades and other events to mark the day. Figures of skeletons in a variety of costumes are a common symbol for *El Día de los Muertos*.

Religion and Culture

In addition to Latinos who are practicing Catholics, it is important for counselors to be aware that many Latinos are "cultural Catholics", meaning that while they may not attend mass or subscribe to all the doctrines of the Catholic Church, they may still find meaning in many of the customs and traditions associated with the religion. For instance, you may meet Latinos who almost never go to church, but when Lent arrives each spring, they are careful not to eat meat on Fridays and instead opt for fish.

Michele

La Virgen de Guadalupe...

While I am not a practicing Catholic, I found comfort and new meaning in the Virgen de Guadalupe as a symbol of a loving and sacrificing mother after my own mother, Guadalupe S. Guzmán, passed away. She was likely named after this patron saint as she was the sole survivor of the seven infants (including her twin) born to my grandmother—as was common in those days, my grandmother had almost no prenatal care and gave birth at home. After my mom's death, I bought a Virgen pendant and candle, and found myself drawn to the symbol that was her namesake.

Another manner in which church doctrine may be weaved into the beliefs of Latinos can be seen in the high Latina teen pregnancy and birth rates.[1] These may be due in part to the views of the Catholic Church on the use of birth control and abortion,[2] and are also likely related to the gender role expectations discussed earlier. In working with young Latinas, a counselor should respectfully explore the messages that they have received regarding sex, sex education, birth control, and abortion. Helping Latinas to negotiate the realities of their sexuality with their faith or cultural adherence to church doctrine may lead to healthier outcomes. Latino culture and the Catholic Church are inextricably linked in many ways.

---

[1] While 34% of girls in the U.S become pregnant at least once as an adolescent, for Latinas this proportion is 51% (The National Campaign to Prevent Teen Pregnancy, 2005).

[2] While the teen pregnancy rate for African Americans is higher than for Latinas, the Latina teen birth rate is the highest among the major racial or ethnic groups in the U.S. because African American teens are more likely to have abortions (Alan Guttmacher Institute, 2004).

FOLK ILLNESSES AND TRADITIONAL HEALING PRACTICES

Among Latinos, there are a variety of folk illnesses. While these may simply seem like Spanish names for illness that are recognized in Western medicine, they are often believed to have spiritual and emotional dimensions as well as natural causes. Illnesses such as *susto* (fright), *nervios* (anxiety), and *empacho* (upset stomach) are common among Latinos who adhere to traditional beliefs (Santiago-Rivera et al., 2002). *Mal de ojo*, often translated as "evil eye", is an example of a belief that supernatural forces can cause illness. It is believed to occur when someone is jealous of another person, or wishes them ill, and stares at the victim and causes sickness to occur. However, mal de ojo may also occur from an admiring stare, and it is believed that a touch from the admiring person will prevent *mal de ojo*. For example, if I see a baby who has beautiful hair, and I stare at the baby's hair in admiration, I have to touch the baby's hair to prevent mal de ojo. Children who get mal de ojo may experience high fever, inability to sleep, and headaches, but mal de ojo is a phenomenon that is not limited to people.

Michele

My grandmother's cactus...

I will never forget the time my grandmother told me that the beautiful cactus she had on her front porch had wilted and died because a relative had given it ojo. It was fine one day, and the next it was shriveled up.

There are a variety of accepted ways to cure *ojo*, which usually involve something along these lines: laying the afflicted person on the floor in a crucifix position and rubbing an egg over the limbs and body while saying the "Our Father" or other prayer. Afterward, the egg is broken and put in a glass of water, and the amount of white or cooked portion is observed (J. L. Garcia, personal communication, December 29, 2005). It may sound strange or funny to those unfamiliar with it, but it is believed to have powerful results.

Regardless of what you believe, it is important to try to understand the client's perspective on his or her illness, regardless of your own beliefs. So much of our experience of illness and healing is what we *believe* about these experiences. This is why you hear drug trial studies talk about "placebo" effects. If someone believes that she will get better, then she probably will feel somewhat better. It is not for us to judge what someone else believes will be healing for him or her. It is most helpful to try to understand how the client conceptualizes the illness: What does the client think caused the illness? What does the client think will help cure the illness or relieve the symptoms? What has the person already tried in treating the illness or in dealing with it? Kleinman (1988, as cited in Fukuyama & Sevig, 2002) calls this "discovering the narrative behind the illness." By working within the client's reality you will get much further in your efforts to heal. It is possible to combine your psychological knowledge and skills with the client's own expertise on his or her experiences to arrive at a successful, collaborative outcome.

Latinos also have their own unique ideas about healing and healers. Latinos with traditional beliefs may seek help from *santeros* (Cubans), *curanderos* (Mexican), and *espiritistas* (Puerto Ricans), who perform rituals using a variety of methods, including lighting candles, saying prayers, and massaging the ill person with special ointments (Santiago-Rivera et al., 2002). These healers may be seen as having more authority than medical doctors and other helping professionals. Therefore, it is important to put our egos aside and work together with other people whom our Latino clients may turn to for help, be they priests, folk healers, or family members. We may find our own doubts getting in the way of believing that traditional ways of healing might be helpful, but we must remember that Indigenous peoples—Mayans, Aztecs, and others—had highly organized and civilized societies before Europeans arrived in the New World. It should be emphasized that not all Latinos may subscribe to the beliefs about folk illnesses and healing outlined here. Many may be perfectly content to rely on Western medical practices, but as already stated it is important to ask a client how he or she conceptualizes the mental or physical illness.

ASSESSING LATINO CLIENTS' ADHERENCE TO CULTURAL NORMS

It has been mentioned throughout this chapter that Latinos will subscribe to cultural norms, traditions, or ideas to a lesser or greater extent based on factors such as generational status, acculturation, education, and socioeconomic status. While some of this information can be obtained directly from intake forms or from acculturation measures (See Santiago-Rivera et al., 2002), much of the assessment regarding this issue can be gained through simply asking the client. This "culturally educated questioning" (Rodriguez & Walls, 2000) is a line of inquiry based on the information you now have about the cultural scripts and practices outlined in this chapter. For instance, with regard to gender roles or familismo, you could ask the client, "What messages have you received about your role in the family?", or "How does your culture influence the way you see your commitment to your family?" In trying to find out if religion is an important part of the client's identity, you might inquire, "What resources do you use to cope with problems?", "From where do you draw strength?", or you might be more specific: "Is religion or spirituality currently an important part of your life?" In seeking a collaborative approach to healing, a counselor might ask, "Are there any cultural practices that you would like to incorporate in our work together?", or "Are there any customs in your culture that might be good for me to know about when thinking about how I might help you?" These are just a few examples of how you might word culturally informed inquires, but hopefully they will provide some guidance for those who are struggling to apply the information presented here to real-life work with clients.

ACCULTURATION

Acculturation, the process of being socialized into a culture other than your own, has in the past been conceptualized as very "either-or." It was thought that a person either remained attached to the native culture, or assimilated entirely into the new host culture. This model was also fairly evaluative and assumed that assimilating was the preferred manner of adaptation. Models then became more complex and multidimensional, recognizing that people may not acculturate as an entire entity, but instead may acculturate to varying extents in different areas of their lives, such as food, dress, language, and values. Finally, these models became bicultural and orthogonal, where it is possible to measure a person's allegiance to their native culture and the new host culture independently. It was recognized that a person could remain attached to their culture of origin to varying degrees and also be acculturated to the dominant society (LaFromboise, Coleman, & Gerton, 1993).

These later, more sophisticated models better account for the reality of many Latinos, who, on a daily basis have to negotiate conflicts between the two cultures. This negotiation is typically stressful and complicated and even with these more complex models, new questions about and perspectives on the conceptualization of acculturation have emerged. For immigrants, there is much to learn in order to be successful in the U.S.: a new language, different cultural norms, and unfamiliar expectations. While migrants likely make choices about which ethnic behaviors and practices they retain, this does not occur in a vacuum, and there may be contextual factors that constrain these choices (Schwartz, Unger, Zamboanga, & Szapocznik, 2010). In examining the changes in how we view acculturation, Schwartz and colleagues (2010) also point out that for some individuals, biculturalism may be more than "simply endorsing both the heritage and receiving cultural streams" (p. 246), but instead may consist of integrating or blending aspects of both cultures into a new cultural experience. They note that there is some evidence that individuals who are able to synthesize the cultures in this way have more positive outcomes such as higher self-esteem, lower psychological distress, and lower acculturation-related stress.

As the theories have improved, so have the measures. At the end of the text, we have included a list of measures that can be used to assess acculturation in Latinos. Because acculturation measures have been around a lot longer than ethnic identity and racial identity development measures, they have worked out many of their early psychometric challenges and have changed to reflect the new multidimensional, orthogonal, bicultural models (Cuéllar, Arnold, & Maldonado, 1995). However, you should still look carefully at the psychometrics of any acculturation measure you choose to use, think about your purpose (research vs. clinical), and be aware of the specific Latino ethnic group you are assessing (as many of the measures have been created for and normed on Mexican-origin populations).

Changing Gender Roles

For both men and women, gender roles may change out of necessity. In order to contribute to the financial support of her family, a woman may have to work outside the home for the first time, leaving less time for the home duties that were previously her responsibility. As a result there is a shifting of these chores to her husband or children. Working outside of the home may also lead to a woman acquiring a new sense of independence and exposure to ideas that run contrary to the more traditional gender role to which some Latinas may have been accustomed; furthermore, a traditional Latino male may feel threatened by these changes in the woman's role. Even for U.S.-born Latinos, acculturation issues around gender roles may be an issue. As the generations progress and Latinos become more acculturated to mainstream European American gender roles, Latinos and Latinas may find themselves moving away from the traditional marianismo and machismo roles presented earlier in this chapter.

Another factor influencing gender roles is the exposure of young people to very sexualized images through music videos, television, movies, and the internet. Young Latinas may feel the pressure between fulfilling expectations from peers and U.S. society and staying true to Latino cultural values concerning the conduct and image of a young woman. All of the gender role changes mentioned here may cause conflict and stress within individuals, couples, and families.

Language Issues

A limited knowledge of English carries with it a number of issues, including limited job opportunities, isolation from others, and general vulnerability when dealing with the society at large, for example, being taken advantage of due to not being able to read documents. Beyond this, however, language issues may be at the core of family dysfunction. Children who come to the U.S. at a young age grow up speaking English and have limited Spanish-speaking skills. This, coupled with parents who have limited English skills, creates a number of problems. It may result in superficial communication between parent and child, thereby stressing their bond. The family hierarchy may be disrupted if children manipulate their parents' access to information from teachers, school officials, and others, or are called upon to be interpreters. Even for Latinos who are not recent immigrants, language may be an issue. Sometimes younger generations are embarrassed to speak Spanish due to fear of discrimination. The flipside of this issue can also be a problem: with increasing frequency, we hear young Latinos say that they wish their parents had taught them Spanish. They feel embarrassed and rejected by other Latinos for not having a command of the language, but usually fail to recognize that their parents did not teach them Spanish to protect them from the discrimination they themselves faced.

Generational Differences

Generational differences between parents and children regarding language and gender roles have been discussed, but other conflicts exist as well. Immigrant or earlier generation parents may hold on to motherland values and culture, whereas their children adopt U.S. cultural norms, resulting in intense conflict. These values may center around familismo. As newer generations acculturate, there may be a greater tendency to put one's individual needs before the family. Conflicts around religion may occur as younger generations leave the Catholic Church or choose to marry outside the faith. Traditions, customs, and food may become lost, forgotten, or devalued. As mentioned earlier, expectations and norms around sex, sexuality, and sexual orientation may change, which is likely to stress the relationships between older and younger generations.

Parenting Issues

In addition to having to cope with children who want more freedom and independence in both behavior and thought, Latino parents must also deal with different expectations regarding parenting in the U.S. There may be a tendency to see educational institutions as fully managing the schooling of their children, thereby leading to a failure by parents to become involved in school functions, conferences, and so on. Documents from the schools may only come in English, thereby limiting parental access to information.

Discipline

An area of serious concern that we have seen in our experiences with Latino clients is the issue of differing expectations around discipline between U.S. society and traditional Latino families, most often with recent immigrants. Corporal (physical) punishment of children is still very much the norm in most Latino countries, and if physical discipline becomes excessive, other family members are usually the ones to intervene. Latino parents may be surprised and confused if Child Protective Services (CPS) becomes involved in discipline issues regarding their children. With an inadequate knowledge of the legal system and a lack of resources to hire legal representation, Latino parents may risk losing custody of their children.

It is very important for a counselor to support Latino families dealing with CPS issues. We are not by any means condoning child abuse, and all counselors are mandated reporters, but we want to stress that taking a supportive and nonjudgmental approach will likely result in more compliance by the parents, and better results. If possible, it is better to have a parent make the call to CPS him or herself to request help if a parenting situation is at a crisis point or if a child's safety is compromised, thereby not further disempowering the client. Additionally, the counselor can do some psychoeducation around differing norms regarding discipline between the U.S. and the client's home country. It is be important to explore the cultural messages the parent has received about discipline, to respect the parent as the expert on his or her child, but also to present alternative disciplinary techniques that are less likely to result in CPS involvement.

AREAS OF RESILIENCY AND STRENGTH

In *Counseling Latinos and la Familia*, Santiago-Rivera, Arredondo, and Gallardo-Cooper (2002) present a list of Latino strengths generated by graduate students in a course entitled Counseling Latinos. The list of strengths includes a worldview that emphasizes unity and cooperation, a pioneer spirit in the face of hardship and structural barriers, and a resiliency grounded in religion and family. Unfortunately, in trying to help counselors-in-training understand the challenges and oppression that Latinos face, a focus on the negative may begin to develop. It's extremely important that we recognize, respect, and make use of the various strengths that Latinos bring to therapy.

Frames of Reference

While it is important to examine the difficulties and barriers that Latinos experience regarding mental illness and access to mental healthcare, it is equally important to recognize the strengths that Latinos bring to counseling. As noted earlier, Latino immigrants tend to have lower rates of mental illness. Suarez-Orozco and Suarez-Orozco (1995) found that Latino immigrant youth used a "dual frame of reference" to help them cope. They used their much more difficult situations in their home countries as a point of comparison when dealing with their current stressors in the U.S. The authors propose that U.S.-born Latinos are more likely to compare their situations to those of their peers in the U.S., see themselves as lacking, and therefore experience more distress. While we would agree that this latter scenario may be true, we would propose that many Latino adults who have now achieved educational and financial success, but had a low SES childhood, may also have this "dual frame of reference". They may be in a better position to appreciate the resources and opportunities they have obtained than peers who have always lived comfortably.

Importance of Family Values

Familismo and the collectivistic sense that Latinos have may also be a strength when dealing with emotional difficulties. Latino families tend to "take care of their own." Therefore, families may act as a safety net or source of support. Additionally, it is likely that extended family will be involved in assisting a Latino individual having difficulty. Grandparents, aunts and uncles, and *madrinas* and *padrinos* (godparents) may all play a role in helping. The video *The Forgotten Americans* (Galan, 2000) presents the plight of Latinos living in *Colonias*, communities formed illegally by unscrupulous developers, where residents live in ramshackle and pieced together houses, often without basic utilities. Henry Cisneros, the narrator of the film, comments that homeless Latinos are rarely seen in the Rio Grande Valley; Latino families would rather live in the deplorable conditions of the Colonias and have some kind of roof over their children's heads than live on the streets.

Michele

My Grandfather's Resourcefulness...

I remember that my grandfather was very resourceful in finding ways to pay for groceries, keep a roof over his and my grandmother's heads, and help my mother, who was a single parent with six kids. He worked as a crossing guard, but would also walk around town collecting aluminum cans and pieces of metal to sell, or would find broken pieces of furniture that people had thrown out, fix them up, and sell them at his almost monthly garage sales. As a self-absorbed adolescent, this seemed almost embarrassing, but now I appreciate the lack of shame he had when it came to being a good provider. Today, I notice that I rarely see Latinos on street corners holding signs asking for money or other assistance; instead I see them busing tables, cleaning bathrooms, picking up garbage, or working hard at some of the other least desirable jobs that our country has to offer. I think that this willingness to work hard and do what has to be done for the sake of one's family is an enormous strength that Latinos possess.

Religion, Spirituality, and Fatalismo

As discussed earlier, religion (usually Catholicism), spirituality, and faith are an important part of Latino culture. We also examined the cultural script of fatalism, and touched on the fact that these cultural norms may be beneficial in many situations. In dealing with mental health issues, there are a variety of ways that such values and beliefs may be helpful. A strong faith in God may provide a sense of hope when dealing with mental illness. The tendency to attribute illnesses and events to external forces or supernatural events may also allow some Latinos to be more tolerant and understanding of those who suffer from emotional ailments. Jenkins (1988) found that many Mexican Americans attributed their relatives' schizophrenia to nervios, a combination of both physical and emotional ailments for which the patient is not to blame, leading the family to be less critical. Family criticism and blame have been associated with relapse in individuals with schizophrenia (Lopez, Nelson, Snyder, and Mintz, 1999, as cited in U.S. Department of Health and Human Services, 2001).

Michele

Si Díos Quiere...

I remember that every time I would say good-bye to my grandparents, they would always say that they would see me the next time "Si Díos quiere," meaning "If God is willing," regardless whether I would be seeing them the next day or months later. I never reflected on this much as a child or adolescent, but in adulthood I came to understand that they really believed exactly what they said. For me, I figured I would pretty much be guaranteed to see them the next time unless I suffered a car accident or some other horrible early demise, but for them, it was not under our control, but up to God. While I support taking our destiny into our own hands, I also can now better appreciate the strength of their viewpoint and beliefs.

There are so many things in this world that we cannot control, and if we hold on to all of them we are likely to feel overwhelmed and anxious. So much of the way we treat anxiety and depression through cognitive therapy is through "reframing," just learning to see things a different way. There is a great amount of strength and wisdom in recognizing that you do not have complete control over whether you will see a loved one the next day, or many other questions in life. Therefore, Latinos' faith in God, fate, luck, or some other higher power should be respected as a strength in dealing with mental health issues and counselors should look for ways to incorporate such resources into treatment.

Biculturalism

All Latinos living in the U.S., including both U.S.-born Latinos and immigrants, have had to face the process of acculturation to some extent. Learning to navigate and negotiate between two cultures is challenging, but also a skill that is developed over time. Many Latinos engage in an "alternation model" of acculturation (LaFromboise, Coleman, & Gerton, 1993), through which they are able to engage in the behaviors, ways of thinking, and other adaptations that are needed to function in their Latino world, but then are able to live, work, and play successfully in a mainstream U.S. culture primarily shaped by European American values. While acculturation stress may be the very problem that brings Latinos to therapy, counselors should point out the ways that clients are already functioning successfully in both worlds. Furthermore, Latinos have a long history of resisting oppression. Indigenous people of the Americas were in one sense "conquered" by the Spaniards and other Europeans, but on the other hand they live on in present day Latino mestizos. I remember being so surprised when I learned that the word that my grandmother used for oatmeal, *atole*, is a word with Aztec roots. I was amazed that elements of Aztec language have survived for hundreds of years and are being spoken by current-day Mexican Americans. While their history and current experience of oppression should be recognized, Latinos should also be conceptualized as survivors.

SUMMARY

This chapter contains a great deal of information about both the ethnic and racial identity development processes, cultural scripts, the resources of Latinos, and the acculturation process. Reading it once will give you some awareness of these issues. We encourage you, as you begin to work with Latinos, to look back over the chapter and see if you are starting to observe these issues coming to life in the experiences of your clients. It is also important that as a developing counselor you explore your own ethnic and racial identity, regardless of your racial and ethnic group membership, and the cultural values that inform how you make sense of the world. Doing so will prepare you to empathize with and understand the identity struggles discussed here that your Latino clients may face. Finally, it may be helpful to think of the ethnic and racial identity development theories, the acculturation process, and the resiliencies that Latinos possess as important knowledge to be integrated with theoretical orientations we practice in the counseling field such as Gestalt, Person-Centered, or Psychodynamic. Doing so will give you tools to employ in helping your Latino clients successfully negotiate identity, cultural, and mental health issues.

CHAPTER 5

Counseling Dynamics and Interventions

INTRODUCTION

This final chapter focuses on therapy interventions and psychological assessment issues in working with Latinos. After an introduction to the outcome research concerning the psychological treatment of Latinos, the issue of premature termination by Latinos in therapy is briefly discussed. Planning effective treatment with Latino clients begins with accurate and careful assessment of their strengths and concerns. Issues related to psychological evaluation are examined in some detail, including the evaluator's cultural competence and language concerns with regard to the tests used and the testing process. Recent literature concerning approaches to counseling Latinos is introduced. Finally, case illustrations are provided, followed by questions and commentary.

LATINO PSYCHOTHERAPY OUTCOME RESEARCH

What do we know about which therapeutic interventions work best for Latino clients? The literature reveals a variety of studies that suggest progress has been made in the psychotherapy outcome research concerning Latinos and other people of color. Altarriba and Bauer (1998) suggest that Hispanics may prefer therapies that have a present-time orientation and ones that are characterized by spontaneous activity and allow for emotional expressiveness. Others have proposed that counseling that allows for active participation by the client in choosing goals and techniques may be helpful because this provides the client with the opportunity to mold the therapy to his or her cultural values (Carrillo, 1978). Furthermore, directive and structured therapies have been suggested for Latinos (Valdes, 1983), especially those who may be of lower socioeconomic status and are in need of rapid symptom relief. Ponterotto (1987) proposed Multimodal Therapy specifically for working with Mexican American clients due to its behavioral and action-oriented nature.

In addition to becoming familiar with the theoretical literature concerning the best way to counsel Latinos, examining the empirical support for such interventions is important. Kanel (2002) collected survey data regarding counseling preferences from 268 low-skilled, low-income laborers as well as college students, all of Mexican descent, living in Southern California. The sample represented different generations and acculturation levels. Both the workers and the students reported a preference for directive, problem-focused therapy approaches. However, the survey only assessed attitudes toward types of therapy, not actual experiences. Rosenthal Gelman (2004) interviewed bilingual/bicultural therapists to evaluate their therapeutic relationships and strategies with Latino clients. The results of this qualitative study indicate that clinicians felt that clients did benefit from psychodynamic therapies, especially when they were modified to reflect a more active and directive approach. Conclusions from this study must be interpreted with caution, as the results are based on the therapists' opinions. While these results also seem to favor a more structured therapeutic approach for Latinos, more research to support this conclusion is needed.

One study that seems to support the need for additional services in conjunction with psychotherapy for some Latinos was an investigation conducted by Miranda, Azocar, Organista, Dwyer, and Areane (2003). These authors conducted a randomized trial that compared cognitive-behavioral group therapy alone, with the same intervention supplemented by clinical case management. The study included seventy-seven Latinos speaking Spanish as their first language; it is notable that all but five of these Latinos were foreign-born. Miranda et al. found lower dropout rates across all racial and ethnic groups for participants receiving case management. However, only participants whose first language was Spanish showed greater improvement in symptoms and functioning than with cognitive-behavioral therapy alone. The combined intervention was actually less effective for those whose first language was English. One limitation to this study is that it does not appear to have included Latino participants whose first language was English. However, what we can learn from this study is that case management services, which included active telephone outreach and working with patients on issues such as housing, employment, and recreation, can make a significant difference in client retention and treatment success for Spanish monolingual immigrant Latinos.

Opler, Ramirez, Dominguez, Fox, and Johnson (2004) found that with Latino patients in need of psychotropic medication, applying a model of cultural sensitivity to the prescription process increased compliance. Working with primarily Dominican patients in the early 1990s at Rafael Tavares Mental Health Clinic in upper Manhattan, these practitioners found that while patients may have been experiencing psychotic symptoms, nerviosismo (anxiety) was their chief complaint. Once physicians stepped away from what they felt were the most salient presenting symptoms (hallucinations) and began treating the anxiety first, they met with increased success. Doctors also had to develop respect for some of these Latino clients' interpretations of hallucinations as spiritual encounters to be valued, not eliminated. The introduction of the antipsychotic medications was done slowly and gradually after initial relief was provided through the anti-anxiety medication. Finally, ongoing education about side effects of the medication proved to be helpful, whereas before the doctors had downplayed such information in fear of making the medication even less palatable. Once these measures were implemented, noncompliance decreased from over 80% to less than 50% within one year. In conjunction with therapy, medication plays a major role in mental health treatment. It is important that psychiatrists, and the psychologists and counselors working together with them, note these important results in making medication delivery more effective for Latino patients.

Further evidence supporting the integration of cultural awareness in the treatment of Latinos and other people of color comes from other studies by Jeanne Miranda and colleagues. Miranda, Schoenbaum, Sherbourne, Duan, and Wells (2004) found that a sample of depressed adults of color, including 258 Latinos, who received "appropriate" care had lower rates of probable depressive disorder (20.5%), compared to 70.5% for those who did not receive it. These participants were receiving individual and group cognitive-behavioral treatment through six managed care organizations across the United States The "appropriate" care for the clients of color included the availability of materials in both English and Spanish, having Latino and African American providers included in videotaped materials, and having information regarding cultural beliefs included in provider training materials. In an investigation of recruiting and retaining low-income Latinos in psychotherapy research, Miranda, Azocar, Organista, Muñoz, and Lieberman (1996) found that using bilingual and bicultural staff, offering services in Spanish, providing transportation, and adding a touch of personalismo increased retention in a number of treatment studies. In one study with high-risk mother–infant dyads, personal warmth was conveyed by monthly phone calls to the participants with attention to details about the participant's situation, birthday cards for mother and baby, and a birthday celebration including cake and a small gift for the child upon completing the study, which occurred on the child's second birthday. Attrition was only 7% in the study of this high-risk group. In the study mentioned earlier, which compared group cognitive-behavioral therapy to this same therapy supplemented with case management (Miranda et al., 2003), investigators were successful at retaining Latinos in the study by calling them the day before each session, and responding to participant concerns that "the treatment was too environmentally cold" (p. 7). In the latter case, the Latino participants were provided coffee and cold drinks during treatment sessions, and were invited to bring food to the final groups to share with others. The investigators found that these adjustments were not necessary in the English-language groups to prevent attrition.

The psychotherapy outcome research presented here points to the importance of both familismo and personalismo in our work with Latino clients. Furthermore, it appears that supplementing cognitive-behavioral intervention with additional services such as outreach and case management can make a difference in the success of treatment of Latinos. Finally, bilingual, bicultural, and culturally competent service providers who can deliver services in Spanish appear to be invaluable to effective treatment.

FACTORS AND ISSUES LEADING TO PREMATURE TERMINATION

For many Latinos who seek therapy, their first contact with a mental health professional is also their last; 50% never return to a psychologist after the first session. By comparison, White individuals drop out at a rate of about 30% (Dingfelder, 2005). Many of the factors that contribute to this issue were examined in Chapter 3: lack of Latino mental health providers, poor health insurance, language barriers, and accessible or convenient facilities. Language tends to be a very significant factor in early termination of counseling.

Nicolás...

I have had many people from Mexico who come to me after they have been referred by their Health Maintenance Organization (HMO) to an English-speaking or limited Spanish-speaking therapist. They report that they were unable to communicate adequately. I once met with a young girl who was unhappy with her therapist. She had requested that the therapist, who was bilingual, speak Spanish when her Spanish, monolingual mother was present. The therapist did not honor her request; in addition to the language barrier, the therapist displayed a lack of respect, and the *confianza* (trust, rapport) was lost. Language and a concomitant lack of adequate communication play a large role in early terminations.

In addition to language difficulties, it has been hypothesized that one reason that ethnic and racial minorities underuse counseling services is that they do not perceive counselors to be competent to address their culturally related concerns. Takeuchi, Sue, and Yeh (1995) found that when ethnic-specific mental health treatment was provided to clients of color, they were more likely to continue treatment beyond one session and to stay for more sessions overall. Fraga, Atkinson, and Wampold (2004) further tested the hypothesis concerning cultural competence on the part of the counselor using a sample of college students that included 152 Latinos. They found that some of the multicultural counseling competencies (MCCs; Sue, Arredondo, and McDavis, 1992) were viewed as more important than others by all participants, but that preference for some MCCs varied depending on the race or ethnicity of the participants. As compared to the White and Asian American students in the sample, one of the MCC preferences most strikingly different for Latinos was the importance placed upon "Understand[ing] the sociopolitical factors that may adversely affect racial/ethnic minorities." This competency was ranked third (out of eleven) by Latino students, whereas Asian American students ranked it eighth, and White students ranked it ninth. While this particular study may only be relevant to college students, and further research is needed, it does tell us that there may be differences in what Latinos find important in their therapist compared with other groups.

ISSUES RELATED TO PSYCHOLOGICAL ASSESSMENT

The psychological assessment of Latino clients has been problematic for decades and it continues to be so. Particularly relevant to a discussion of this issue is a long-standing history of using "standardized" psychological instruments to assess Latino clients. These instruments, however, were standardized using European American samples, and their use resulted in frequent misdiagnoses of Latino clients as having mental retardation or learning disabilities. The misuse of standardized instruments was particularly rampant in the 1960s and 1970s. Although there is much greater awareness of the problem today, it still exists to the same, if not a greater, degree. In the past, test developers did not include Latinos in their samples, whereas today they take care to include Latinos and other diverse populations in their samples. However, the numbers are so small that it appears test-developers may merely be paying lip service to the issue of cross-cultural validity. Psychologists may get fooled into thinking that because Latinos were included in the sample they can therefore use the instrument and not have to take into account cultural factors. Furthermore, many psychologists take for granted that because Latino individuals were included in the sample, they themselves do not have to be knowledgeable about Latino culture in order to make a valid interpretation of the results. Similarly, test developers are now cognizant of the growing market of Spanish-language psychological instruments, and in the haste to fill that need they have translated instruments into Spanish. On the one hand, the fact that more Spanish language instruments are available is a tremendous improvement over just a decade ago, but as will be discussed below, this too has its problems. In sum, most psychologists today are well aware that issues of cross-cultural applicability and validity of psychological instruments are important. However, we have been lulled into a false sense of comfort regarding this issue, making the misuse of instruments just as likely today as forty years ago. Today, we recognize two main factors as problematic: lack of cross-culturally valid instruments and lack of cultural competence on the part of the examiner.

Cross-Cultural Validity of Instruments

Efforts to address the cross-cultural validity of instruments have been growing over the last decade or two. Some of the major instruments now have versions in Spanish or at least instructions for administering the instrument in Spanish. A review of the *PsychCorp*™ Annual Catalogue (2006) reveals more than a dozen instruments available in Spanish, from intelligence tests to neuropsychological instruments to observation rating forms and self-report forms for emotional states. The percentage of tests in Spanish, however, remains small when compared to the number of English-language instruments.

The advantage of having Spanish-language instruments available is that administration of the instrument is standardized. This is certainly a vast improvement over past practice, when English-speaking examiners would read aloud the items of the test being administered and the items would then be translated by a Spanish-speaking aide. Alternatively, Spanish-speaking examiners would translate an instrument from English to Spanish as they were administering the instrument, making each administration different from the next. The psychologist whose practice included a good number of Spanish-language clients would translate (for himself/herself) available instruments, to facilitate and somewhat standardize the administration process. This was "best practice" just a few years ago, and in many cases continues to be. This certainly has its problems, as clearly identified by Hambleton and Pastula (1999), including not only the lack of linguistic equivalence, but also lack of construct equivalence, which would completely invalidate both the test and the results.

A standardized administration improves the reliability of the instrument, but it does nothing to address its utility and validity. A psychologist who is well versed in test development and knowledgeable about issues of cross-cultural equivalence in instrument development will readily spot significant problems with most Spanish-language psychological instruments developed in the U.S. Translations are done with little regard for cultural factors. For example, while it is easy enough to translate the question "What are the colors of the American flag?" into Spanish, that question does not have the same meaning for a child born and raised in Guatemala as it does for a child born and raised in the United States. The same would be true for most other questions on the "information" subtest on an intelligence test developed in the United States. Similarly, it is easy enough to translate the instructions on a "performance" or "nonverbal" subtest (like *Block Design* or *Object Assembly)*, but there is no way to equate the cultural experience of a child born and raised in a middle-class family in the United States (where there has been easy access to blocks and puzzles) with that of a child born and raised in a *ranchito* (village) in Mexico.

To add to the problem, it is not uncommon to find that translations are poorly done; one frequently finds that key words are translated literally, and although the translation is literally accurate there tends to be a slight shift in the concept being tested or in the meaning of the phrase. There is the additional concern that, in the United States, many Latinos are bilingual, and that poses a different problem. As Kester and Peña (2002) report, Spanish/English bilingual language development differs significantly from monolingual language development, and testing a bilingual individual in either English or Spanish only will not sufficiently allow for full expression of what the individual knows. Thus, simply having a Spanish-language instrument will not suffice for accurate assessment of English/Spanish bilinguals. In sum, one of these factors alone might be enough to cause significant error of measure for someone from a different culture; in combination, they will completely invalidate the results.

Finally, although a Spanish-language instrument will help with standardized administration, it does nothing to address the lack of appropriate norms. Most psychological instruments that have been translated into Spanish do not have corresponding norms derived from Spanish-speaking samples. There are some instruments that have been normed in Spain (for example the Wechsler Adult Intelligence Scale-III), but Spain is in Europe, and although the language might be the same, the cultural experience is vastly different from that of Latinos in the Western Hemisphere. Compared to three or four decades ago, when Spanish-language psychological instruments were almost non-existent, there has been tremendous progress in the field, resulting in the availability of many Spanish-language instruments (see Resource List). The availability of such instruments makes possible standardized, reliable administration, but as indicated above, issues of validity remain largely unresolved. For that reason, it is important for the examiner to be knowledgeable about cross-cultural testing issues; in addition, the examiner should be familiar with Latino culture, as will be discussed below.

Cultural Competence of the Examiner

A psychologist working with Latino clients, especially Spanish-speaking Latino clients, may find some Spanish-language instruments to facilitate the assessment of bilingual or monolingual Spanish-speaking clients. However, it will be much more difficult to find all the valid instruments needed to conduct a *comprehensive* psychological assessment. For that reason, when working with Latino populations the psychologist is his or her own best instrument. In this respect, in order to make full use of oneself as a psychological instrument one must be a culturally competent psychologist. Professionally, cultural competence refers to one's ability to provide culturally relevant services to clients from diverse cultures. When evaluating Latino clients there are a number of issues that must be taken into account if one is to provide culturally competent services. The extent to which these issues are pertinent depends on your own level of acculturation, bilingualism, and biculturalism, as well as the client's. In order to assess whether an evaluation was conducted in a culturally competent manner, a number of questions might be asked.

Evaluator's Education and Training

The evaluator should be familiar with cross-cultural testing issues by virtue of education or supervised work. The following questions serve as a guideline to assess your own (or someone else's) level of cultural competence for assessing Latino clients. These are basic or minimum requirements.

- Did the evaluator take graduate courses in cross-cultural psychology that include directly working with clients from diverse cultures, or testing culturally diverse clients? If not, has the evaluator taken continuing education courses in these areas?
- Is the evaluator cognizant of issues of fairness in testing people of color or clients from diverse cultures?
- Is the evaluator familiar with how or to what extent a particular test used during the evaluation may be culturally biased?
- In testing a client from a different culture, did the evaluator do the "standard" evaluation (the same instruments that she uses with all clients), or did the evaluator take into account the client's background before selecting the tests used?
- If tested in a language other than English, was a standardized translation employed? If not, did the evaluator address this issue in his interpretation of the results?

Evaluator's knowledge and use of the language

In order to conduct a competent psychological evaluation of a Latino client, one must be familiar with the particular dialect of Spanish the client speaks. Degree of cultural competence will vary depending on the evaluator's knowledge, use, and facility with Spanish. In the U.S., a large percentage of cases that are referred for testing involve clients with limited formal Spanish; they primarily speak a dialect, so it is important to be familiar with vernacular as well as formal Spanish. The following are basic questions to ask when assessing competence.

- Does the evaluator know the language?
- Where did the evaluator learn the language? Is that location different from where the client learned it? (Spanish learned in the classroom differs significantly from vernacular.)
- How often does the evaluator practice speaking the language, and in what context(s)?
- Is the evaluator familiar with a variety of vernacular or colloquial expressions?

Use of an Interpreter

In the U.S. there is currently a great need for Spanish-speaking psychologists which will probably not be met anytime soon. As was the case forty years ago, some psychologists will use interpreters to conduct psychological evaluations. When this is the situation, answering the following basic questions will help assess the degree to which the evaluation was conducted in a culturally competent manner.

- Who was the interpreter? (Be aware that family members, friends, or others who work with the client may be invested in a certain outcome.)
- Is she or he a certified translator?
- What is the extent of the interpreter's medical or psychological training?
- To what extent is the interpreter familiar with psychological and medical terms and expressions?

Evaluator's Knowledge of the Culture

Finally, the evaluator's knowledge of Latino culture will impact his or her ability to conduct a psychological evaluation with cultural competence. Simply knowing the language is not enough to properly interpret the results of psychological instruments or techniques, including the clinical interview. There are nuances of Latino culture that can easily be misinterpreted as symptoms of severe psychopathology if one is unfamiliar with them. A few of these (some of which were discussed in Chapter 4) include believing in spirits, *brujeria,* and santeria, and ailments like *mal de ojo*, as well as cultural elements such as family unity, cooperation, interdependence and strongly bonded parent-child dyads. All these can be misinterpreted if one is not familiar with the culture. To assess if the evaluator is culturally competent, one might ask to what extent she or he is familiar with the significance of Latino cultural elements. For example, is the examiner familiar with the difference in family structure and dynamics between mainstream U.S. and Latino families? This includes the significant role played by *abuelos* (grandparents) and extended relatives such as aunts, uncles, and cousins, in addition to figurative extended relatives like madrinas and padrinos (godparents) and *comadres* and compadres. In addition, the examiner should be familiar with basic rituals, like *bautizos* (Baptism), *quinceañeras* (fifteenth birthday celebrations), and some courtship and marriage practices. The evaluator should be familiar with basic foods and how they are prepared, and should know some of the more important holidays and their meanings, such as *Día de los Reyes* (January 6th), *Semana Santa* (Holy Week), *Cinco de Mayo* (May 5th), *Dieciséis de Septiembre* (September 16th), *Día de los Muertos* (November 1st), and *Día de la Virgen de Guadalupe* (December 12th). It would also help to know a little about important art and artists, literature, and some prominent heroes and personalities, and it is important to keep up with—at least—the headlines of current events that affect or involve Latinos in areas like politics, government, and immigration.

In addition to being familiar with the cultural elements listed above, it is important for a psychologist to be familiar with the nuances of Latino cultural reality and how it differs from U.S. cultural reality, especially regarding concepts presented on the following table.

LATINO versus U.S. CULTURAL REALITY

European American	Latino
Education	**Knowledge**
Credentials	Wisdom
Expertise	**Experience**
Status	Place
Success	Accomplishment
Performance	Fulfillment of duty
Physical	**Spiritual**
Curing	Healing
Quack	Curandero
Suffering	Sacrifice
Relatedness	**Relationship**
Individual	Family
Nuclear Family	Extended Family
Neutrality	Empathy
Husband–Wife dyad	Parent–child dyad
Assimilation	**Enculturation**
Monolingualism	Bilingualism
Monoculturalism	Biculturalism

It must be cautioned that generational status in the U.S. and level of acculturation across various dimensions must be taken into account when determining the cultural "reality" or norms to which a Latino individual subscribes. The evaluator who is knowledgeable about and actively seeks out opportunities to engage and interact with Latinos and their culture will be much better prepared to conduct a culturally relevant and valid psychological assessment.

APPROACHES TO COUNSELING LATINOS

As with psychological assessment, the counseling of Latino clients has had its problems. Traditional approaches to therapy are based on European and European American theory and practice, making them potentially ill-suited for use with Latinos, many of whom have Indigenous and African ancestry. In addition, nuances of Latino culture are at odds with the "blank slate" approach to therapy and with the maintenance of rigid boundaries recommended in the guidelines and principles espoused by most counseling and psychological organizations. Psychological theory is simply that: theory, a guide for understanding behavior, not a rigid set of rules. Ethical guidelines and principles do not quite have the mandate of law, but in practice most psychologists follow them to the letter. It is a system that works well in the U.S because it fits with, and was developed for, this culture (See the table on Latino versus U.S. cultural reality above). The system is quite lacking, however, when applied to Latinos. Latinos are a warm, inviting people, who are very connected to the community. As is evidenced by the psychotherapy outcome research presented above, when they need and seek help, Latinos do not want to go see a stranger, they want to see someone they know or someone that their family or friends know. They do not look for rigid boundaries; they look for a relationship. They do not want to see credentials or someone who espouses theory; they want someone who will make them feel welcome and who will impart wisdom. They want to be warmly received and to hear their own language, and it is as important for them to know where their therapist or counselor is from as it is to know what the therapist or counselor does. Thus, when working with Latino clients, one must be more willing to respond to questions of a personal nature and to engage in *platica* (chat or small talk) with one's clients.

Nicolás...

Some of the literature suggests that Latinos are ignorant about the role of psychologists and other mental health professionals, but in my experience, having worked with hundreds of Spanish-speaking clients from Mexico and various other Latin American countries with varying degrees of education, I have never been asked what I do. Almost invariably, however, I am asked where I am from and where I learned Spanish. Latino clients never ask where I have studied. By contrast, European American clients often ask about my degree. For Latinos the connection to community and the culture is more important than my education and my credentials. Knowing this, and being comfortable answering those questions, promotes rapport with Latino clients.

While it is important to address Latino adult clients formally, using *"usted"* rather than the informal *"tu,"* it is also important to be casual in conversation and to use platica in the sessions. One must be willing to allow some give-and-take in the relationship rather than maintaining strict boundaries, and at times there may be a need for the counselor or psychologist to step out of that role and serve as an advocate for the client. This permits the counselor to become a *persona de confianza* (trustworthy person), cementing the relationship. However, we are warned against these practices by our ethical guidelines and principles. It is the task of the psychologist to learn to navigate the fine line between ethical principles and guidelines and cultural competence, which will promote the therapeutic relationship with Latino clients.

Language Switching

Throughout this text we have emphasized the importance of language in working with Latinos. The case for bilingual service providers and therapy offered in Spanish has been made and is supported by research. Here, we would like to mention ways in which language can be used therapeutically (Santiago-Rivera, 1995; Santiago-Rivera and Altarriba, 2002). People typically store memories in their minds in the language in which the event occurred. For that reason, if the goal is to have a client connect more closely with the emotional content of an event, it should be done in the language in which the incident is "programmed." For this reason, even when working with Latinos who are bilingual, it may be helpful for them to "switch" into the language needed to more fully explore a past issue or problem. The same can be said of working on relationships or communication. If a client is having a problem with an elderly parent and the communication with that parent occurs in Spanish, it may be helpful to work on the issue in Spanish. In the same way that language can be used to assist a client in more closely exploring an issue, switching away from the language in which a traumatic event occurred may enable a client to more safely explore the event in the initial stages of therapy.

Storytelling (*Cuentos*) and Sayings (*Dichos*)

Another manner in which to provide culturally sensitive therapy to Latinos is through storytelling and Spanish proverbs. Costantino, Malgady, and Rogler (1986) developed and empirically investigated *cuento* therapy, the use of cultural folktales and storytelling as a therapeutic intervention for use with Latino children. Cuento therapy has been shown to enhance the development of ethnic identity and pride, and to educate individuals about cultural values and standards of behavior (Costantino and Rivera, 1994, as cited in Santiago-Rivera et al., 2002). In their study of 210 first- to third-grade Puerto Rican children demonstrating maladaptive behaviors, they compared the use of cuentos from Puerto Rican culture that modeled adaptive behaviors, with traditional art/play therapy, and no therapy. They found that the cuento therapy was superior to the other approaches and significantly reduced trait anxiety, even one year later.

Dichos are Spanish sayings or proverbs that capture popular wisdom. Because all Latinos use sayings, metaphors, and similes in their everyday conversation, these sayings are widely available to bring into the counseling experience. Dichos are powerful because of their rich imagery and meaning, and because Latinos often communicate ideas in an indirect or subtle manner

(Santiago-Rivera, et al., 2002). Dichos may be a useful way of exploring topics in therapy that are difficult to breach in a more direct fashion. Zúñiga (1992) was one of the first practitioners to explore the effectiveness of using dichos in therapy. She demonstrated the use of dichos in reducing client resistance, reframing problems, and increasing motivation. If you are unfamiliar with dichos, you may check the web site *Del Dicho al Hecho* (Esteban Giménez) listed in our resource list at the end of the book, or simply ask clients for common sayings used by family or friends that they have found helpful.

The Family Coping Skills Program: An Example of Treatment Infused with Cultural Awareness

The outcome research presented earlier demonstrates that some researchers and practitioners are trying to incorporate sensitivity to Latino cultural values into treatment interventions. Cardemil, Kim, Pinedo, and Miller (2005) designed the Family Coping Skills Program (FCSP), a culturally appropriate mental health intervention designed to prevent depression in low-income Latina mothers. The group sessions, which formed the base of the program, were cognitive-behavioral in nature. A family meeting component was built into the program in recognition of the importance of familismo in Latino culture, and also because of the strong evidence that family members play a role in the development and maintenance of depression. Other culturally sensitive aspects of the training included flexibility with regard to the language in which treatment was received (English or Spanish); culturally relevant material in the sessions (topics regarding immigration, acculturation, and discrimination); and culturally competent group leaders (familiar with Latino culture and bilingual). Childcare, bus passes, and taxi vouchers were also provided to facilitate participant attendance. While the conclusions that can be drawn from the first thirty-three participants are preliminary, they point toward the potential success of the program. Over 70% of the participants engaged in the treatment study attended at least four group sessions (out of six) and there was a statistically significant decrease in the mean Beck Depression Inventory scores of these completers, representing a mean reduction of 36% of symptoms from pre- to post-intervention. While more research is needed, results such as these from programs carefully designed to meet the needs of Latinos are encouraging.

CASE ILLUSTRATIONS
Child Protection and Parenting Issues

A "Mentally Retarded" Woman
Child Protective Services (CPS) removed children from the home following allegations of neglectful supervision and physical abuse. Subsequently the mother, a native of Mexico, submitted to a psychological evaluation conducted by a European American psychologist who spoke limited Spanish

(continues)

CASE ILLUSTRATIONS *(continued)*

and who was unfamiliar with Mexican culture. In his evaluation, the psychologist found indicators that the mother may have suffered some significant trauma, and diagnosed her with Post-Traumatic Stress Disorder. Using a standardized intellectual screening instrument which consisted of the administration of four subtests, the psychologist found the mother (and the father) to have limited intellectual capabilities, diagnosed her with Mild Mental Retardation, and suggested that the mother was not the best candidate to be the primary caregiver for her children. The mother disputed the results of the evaluation, and the CPS caseworker referred her for an evaluation with a psychologist who was fluent in Spanish and familiar with Mexican culture; the psychologist conducted the entire evaluation in Spanish.

During the first meeting, the mother entered the examiner's office readily and without hesitation. She easily provided identifying information, and she understood and signed the *Consent for Release of Information* form. However, she seemed unable to understand the *Consent for Evaluation* form, not comprehending, as stated on the form, that the results of the psychological evaluation "might support her goal of regaining custody of her children, or they might show evidence to the contrary." She seemed unable to conceive or understand the possibility that her children may not be returned to her, even though this was explained orally by the examiner five or six times. Furthermore, it seemed obvious that she was quite unfamiliar with and quite confused by the entire process of CPS intervention, the psychological evaluation, and the legal possibilities. The psychologist stopped the testing process, and recommended that the mother consult with her attorney.

After consulting with her attorney, the mother returned to complete the evaluation. During the course of the evaluation, she explained to the examiner that during the previous evaluation, she was simply "told to do this and do that," but she never understood the purpose or the process of the evaluation. During the evaluation with the Spanish-speaking psychologist, the mother was quite verbal and able to clearly express her opinions. She was spontaneous and spoke in a firm and clear voice. She was appropriately assertive and was the primary contact person for the examiner throughout the evaluation process (of her husband and herself). The allegations and history on record and the results of the previous evaluation were reviewed with the mother. She denied or minimized the seriousness of allegations stated in the record, which indicated that:

- There was not always enough food in the house.
- The children did not have much clothing and their shoes were tattered and worn.
- The mother left the children in the care of her brother, who had spent four months in a psychiatric hospital and had been diagnosed with schizophrenia.
- The mother had lost two children in Mexico; one had drowned in a river and the other had died after being attacked by a wild animal.

(continues)

CASE ILLUSTRATIONS *(continued)*

The mother stated that what was in the records were "all lies" made up by the CPS worker. For example, she indicated that she always had plenty of food for her children, and that they were always well dressed and clean. She indicated that her brother had been in the hospital "because he stopped eating," but disavowed awareness that he may have more serious pathology. She acknowledged that her first two children had died, but indicated that one had drowned in a stream while in the care of one of her sisters. The second child had been medically fragile since birth and had died despite having been treated regularly by physicians in major cities in Mexico and having spent one month in hospital.

The mother reported to the examiner that she and her husband were from a small village in southern Mexico where there was no running water or electricity. She and her husband had traveled over 1000 miles to reach the United States; they had lived here about seven years before sending for their children, who had lived with them about three years before the alleged incident of neglect. All members of the family remain undocumented. The mother reported that she had never attended school, but since coming to the U.S. she had taught herself to read and write Spanish at a rudimentary level. She acknowledged to this examiner that her husband had been arrested and incarcerated for almost two months for driving while intoxicated (something she did not report in the previous evaluation), and that it was during his incarceration that the children had been removed.

In Deciding How to Respond to this Case, Consider:

- What are some reasons an examiner unfamiliar with Mexican culture might consider this woman to be a person with mental retardation?
- What might an examiner familiar with Mexican culture consider as evidence that this woman is not mentally retarded?
- What might help you determine whether a culturally competent evaluation had been performed by either examiner?
- How do you account for the woman's different presentation with the Spanish-speaking psychologist after speaking with her attorney?
- What cultural elements might an examiner have to consider or be familiar with in order to make an appropriate assessment in this case?
- What might be appropriate recommendations for this case?

Response and Recommendation   The use of a valid measure of intelligence in this case will be critical. While one might use a "nonverbal" measure of intelligence, one must keep in mind that the client and her husband were born and raised in a village in Mexico; they have no formal education and they have lived a rudimentary lifestyle the better part of their lives. In this case the examiner felt that the best instrument to use to assess intelligence level was the EIWA (*Escala de Inteligencia de Wechsler para Adultos*), even though it is outdated. The EIWA was developed in the 1960s and

CASE ILLUSTRATIONS *(continued)*

normed in Puerto Rico on adults with little formal education. It was used in this case because the norm sample was more similar to the client than norm samples of more recent instruments. Even "nonverbal" tests, which are often considered "culture-free," are heavily biased in favor of a middle-class lifestyle.

In cases of mental retardation, it is important to compare the individual's adaptive functioning with the results of intelligence testing. This woman and her husband traversed 1000 miles to arrive in the United States. They had worked for over ten years to support themselves and their children. She had taught herself to read and write, albeit at an elementary level. The woman and her husband arrived at the examiners office using the bus system. She was able to explain how to cook complex meals like *enchiladas* and *chiles rellenos*, and could explain how to wash and iron clothing. She and her husband paid bills and had never been evicted from a house or apartment.

The client and her husband both scored in the Average range of intelligence on the EIWA. Based on the results of the EIWA and assessment of adaptive function, it was the examiner's opinion that neither the client nor her husband was mentally retarded. It was clear that this family lived in poverty, but poverty is not neglect. America is a nation of immigrants and the vast majority of first generation immigrants live in poverty; their children usually fare better. The best way to assess neglect and abuse of a child is to assess the child, not the parent. It was recommended that the children be assessed by a Spanish-speaking psychologist to determine whether there had been abuse before deciding on the appropriate intervention for the family.

Catch-22

Mr. and Mrs. M, ages 26 and 24, are middle-class Costa Rican immigrants. They came to the U.S. on a visitor visa, which they decided to overstay in order to work and save some money before returning home. During the course of their stay, Mrs. M became pregnant, and they had their first and only child. When the child was about four months old, he was taken to the hospital to be treated for a fractured leg. The parents report that the mother was holding the child when the child slipped out of her arms, and she grabbed the child by the leg to prevent him from hitting the floor. Subsequently, full-body X-rays revealed that the child had several fractures that were at various stages of healing, including his toes and several ribs. Both parents denied having injured the child, but both were suspected of abuse and were asked to participate independently in "Protective Parenting Classes," in which they were unsuccessful because neither was willing to either admit to abuse or to believe and acknowledge that the other parent had injured the child. They were treated by two different therapists with varying degrees of fluency in Spanish. Mr. M, in particular, complained of problems communicating with his therapist.

(continues)

CASE ILLUSTRATIONS *(continued)*

Since neither parent acknowledged having hurt the child, nor believed that the other parent might have injured the child, they were considered treatment failures and therefore could not regain custody of the child, and were referred for counseling. Both parents presented as intelligent, assertive individuals. They each made good eye contact and spoke in a firm audible voice. Both Mr. and Mrs. M report having been raised in healthy family environments by loving parents. Criminal background checks did not reveal antisocial history of either parent in the U.S. or in Costa Rica. There was no history of alcohol or drug use, and no history of domestic violence.

In Deciding How to Respond to this Case, Consider:
- What role did language play in Mr. and Mrs. M's treatment?
- How might have a lack of confianza (trust, rapport) played a factor in Mr. and Mrs. M's treatment failure?
- What cultural elements, such as familismo, marianismo, and machismo, might have played a role in neither person confessing to abusing the child?
- How do you think their undocumented status might have factored into the couple's reluctance to admit the abuse?
- What possible recommendations could be made in this case for the safety and well-being of the child?

Response and Recommendation   Both of these clients were facing possible criminal charges of a very serious nature, and were both acutely aware of this issue. Their undocumented status put them at further legal risk. They had agreed to return to Costa Rica, but if either one had admitted to the abuse, they would likely have faced prosecution in the U.S. Therefore, if they had not yet confessed to hurting the child, it was unlikely that they were going to do so with the new therapist. It is important to keep roles clear. While psychologists and counselors are mandated reporters of abuse, it is not their job to investigate such abuse. In previous treatment, the objective had been to get the clients to confess to hurting the child or admit that the spouse had injured the child. Knowledge of the importance of the parent–child bond in Latino families led the new therapist to shift the treatment objective. Rather than trying to elicit a confession or acknowledgment of hurting the child, the new therapist made the safety of the child the treatment objective, something on which all parties could agree.

Language was also an issue in this case. Mr. M felt uncomfortable with the language ability of his previous therapist, but more important was the issue of trust, as the previous therapists and the clients were working at cross-purposes. Knowledge of the language facilitated trust with Mr. M. After discussion of family histories with both clients, the therapist recommended that the child be placed with family members in Costa Rica, and that the case be transferred to the Costa Rican equivalent of Child

(continues)

CASE ILLUSTRATIONS *(continued)*

Protective Services. Knowing that Costa Rica is one of the wealthiest countries in Latin America gave confidence that services would be available for the child and the family in that country, ensuring the safety of the child.

"EN MI CASA, NO" (NOT IN MY HOME)

Leti, a 14-year-old Puerto Rican girl, attempted to hurt herself and was taken to the local psychiatric hospital. The mother reported to hospital staff that Leti was *endemoniada* (possessed by the devil), and during the course of taking a social history it was discovered that her mother was encouraging Leti to date a 21-year-old man. Therefore, CPS became involved, removed Leti from her home, and she was referred for treatment.

Leti was brought to the interview by her foster parents, who were an English-speaking lesbian couple. Leti is bilingual, though she is more comfortable speaking Spanish. During her interview, Leti reported that she is a native of Puerto Rico, and that she has been in the U.S. only a few months. She reported a relatively normal developmental history. Leti also shared that she was a lesbian, and that in Puerto Rico, she was "dating" and having sexual contact with a 22-year-old woman. Leti indicated that her mother was opposed to this relationship and to her being a lesbian, which is the reason that they came to the U.S. The mother was seen separately, and her report was consistent with Leti's reported developmental history and the reasons for coming to the U.S. The mother stated that she had encouraged Leti's relationship with the 21-year-old man, who was a friend of the family, so that Leti would forget about the woman she had been "dating" in Puerto Rico. She also stated that she could not accept Leti's sexual orientation, and that she would not have her live in her home if she was going to chose to be with women.

In Deciding How to Respond to this Case, Consider:

- How might Latino gender roles, and marianismo in particular, play a part in the mother's view of Leti's sexual orientation?
- How religion and spirituality are informing Leti's mother's understanding of her daughter's sexual orientation?
- How might Leti's living in a home with a lesbian couple affect the outcome of this case, given the mother's views?
- How might you help both Leti and her mother understand the differences in sexual behavior norms (regarding children and adults) in Puerto Rico versus the U.S.?
- How might you help Leti and her mother better understand and respect the other's position?
- What might "success" look like in this case?

Response and Recommendation

Several issues are at play in this case. In order to assess the degree of pathology in this family, one must be familiar

(continues)

CASE ILLUSTRATIONS *(continued)*

with Puerto Rican norms/values regarding the sexual behavior of both juveniles and adults, religious norms, gender issues, and family relationships. In this case, things became complicated by placement of the child with a lesbian, English-speaking couple, for several reasons. The mother saw this as a double betrayal by the system and an undermining of her parental authority. She thus lost complete trust in anyone connected with that system, including the therapist, and she was not willing to accept the therapist's recommendations, which included speaking with a priest and reading materials written by lesbian Latina authors.

Leti, while happy to be away from her mother, became more conflicted. Despite their problems, she loved her mother, but the foster parents tended to vilify the mother for her beliefs and were more interested in supporting the child's sexual orientation than in helping her resolve the conflict with her mother. Two years after being referred for treatment, the child was still in foster care, and the relationship with her mother remained strained.

Sexual Behavior Problems

My Brother, My Son

Mr. G came from Mexico over twenty years ago, and as soon as he was able became a legal resident of the U.S. He subsequently arranged to bring his children and his wife to join him; they are now also legal residents of the U.S., have adjusted well, and are currently living a lower-middle class lifestyle. Mr. and Mrs. G's older children completed high school in the U.S. and all currently work in construction. The youngest child, José, is the adopted son of Mr. and Mrs. G., but biologically José is Mr. G's half-brother, the product of a union between Mr. G's father and his second wife. Mr. and Mrs. G reported that José's biological mother was emotionally unstable; she unsuccessfully attempted to terminate her pregnancy with José on more than one occasion, and after his birth attempted to hurt him. When José was about six months old, she abandoned him in a field, where he was found crying. It was at that point that the elder Mr. G asked his son and daughter-in-law to adopt and raise José.

José has no significant medical problems, but he has been diagnosed with Attention Deficit/Hyperactivity Disorder (ADHD) and is being treated by his family physician for this condition. He currently takes Ritalin, 10mg in the morning; he has been on the same dosage for three years. José manifested behavioral problems in school from an early age, which continued even after he started taking ADHD medication. José readily admits that he has difficulties with teachers and classmates. His parents are also aware of this but seemed at a loss as to how to help José; they trusted that the medication would suffice in ameliorating the problems. It did not, however, and José now finds himself almost 13 years old and in the fifth grade. He also has had some behavior problems (making a false 911 call) for which he was placed on probation, and he is currently charged with sexual

(continues)

CASE ILLUSTRATIONS *(continued)*

assault, a charged levied by his 12-year-old girlfriend's mother. Because of all the behavioral problems José is having, his parents are debating whether they should inform José about his birth history and give him the choice of going to live with his biological father in Mexico or staying with them here in the U.S., where he was raised and where his older adoptive brothers live.

Mr. and Mrs. G do not speak English, but José is fully bilingual. José was assessed, by court order, by an English-speaking psychologist, who concluded that José was "dangerous" and needed to be incarcerated. As a result, José was placed under "house arrest" while awaiting trial. The parents sought out a Spanish-speaking examiner and requested a new evaluation. The Spanish-speaking examiner conducted a bilingual assessment. The interview with Mr. and Mrs. G was conducted entirely in Spanish. José's interview and assessment were conducted in both English and Spanish, depending on which he was most comfortable with. Most of the interview was conducted in Spanish, with occasional use of English, while most of the testing was conducted in English with occasional use of Spanish. During testing, the examiner noticed that although José first responded to the item in English, he often switched to Spanish at the end of his comment to clarify or more fully explain his response.

In Deciding How to Respond to this Case, Consider:

- What are some reasons an English-speaking examiner might consider José to be "dangerous" and in need of incarceration?
- How might using a Spanish-speaking examiner benefit José?
- What might help you determine whether a culturally competent evaluation had been performed by either examiner?
- How does the cultural value of familismo figure into this case?
- Is it possible that José might be experiencing discrimination at school or elsewhere? How so?
- Do you have any concerns about the status of José's medication and diagnosis?
- How might you advocate for José? In what areas does he need advocacy?

Response and Recommendation   The prominent issues in this case are advocacy for the client and bilingual/biculturalism. When they become involved in the legal system, Latino clients are often referred to a psychologist, most of whom are English-speaking and have a contract with the courts to provide assessment services. This limits the possibility of a client who is in jeopardy of being incarcerated getting a valid assessment. When the referral is made, Latino clients who are unfamiliar with the system often simply do as they are told by court officers, fully trusting that they will be treated fairly. Unfortunately, they often are not. In cases such as this, the culturally competent psychologist hired by the family must not

(continues)

CASE ILLUSTRATIONS *(continued)*

only perform the assessment, but may also need to act as an advocate for the client to ensure that he is being treated fairly.

Because they are fluent in English, bilingual children are often referred for and assessed completely in English, without much thought given to whether the results of the assessment are valid. José's case clearly demonstrates the importance of permitting bilingual individuals the opportunity to express themselves in both languages. After giving an English response, José added further information in Spanish, making a big difference in the information that he provided. The English-speaking psychologist did not have the benefit of this additional material, so his results were based on incomplete information, resulting in his conclusion that José was highly dangerous. In the bilingual evaluation, José still demonstrated problems, but not dangerousness. A term of probation with outpatient treatment was recommended.

Incest

When he was 14 years old, Manuel was arrested and charged with the sexual abuse of his niece. He was released to the custody of his sister to await trial, but he absconded to Mexico. He returned to the United States about a year later, was arrested again, and remained incarcerated at the time of the referral. He was referred for assessment by the juvenile authorities, who also wanted an evaluation regarding his risk for fleeing the country and recommendations for treatment. The interview and assessment were conducted entirely in Spanish.

Manuel is a 15-year-old boy born and raised in a small ranchito (village) in Mexico, where his parents still live. The rest of his family (two brothers and three sisters) currently live in the U.S., not far from the Mexican border. Although they have been in the U.S. for over twelve years, all his family members remain undocumented. Manuel is the youngest of the siblings; he had been coming to the U.S. off-and-on for about three years before he took up permanent residence with his youngest sister and his brother-in-law, who serve as his guardians.

Manuel was raised in a stable and loving family environment. The siblings are close to each other, and the family members count on each other for help. Except for the father becoming easily angered and "yelling," no history of family dysfunction is reported. Manuel also denied a history of any type of abuse or of having witnessed family violence, though when he was about 10 years old, he himself was sexually abused by an older cousin. There is no history of antisocial activity by any of the family members, all of whom work in construction, although they have been known to occasionally get into physical altercations.

Manuel has no history of serious illness, head injuries, or hospitalizations. He has always performed well academically. He had no behavioral difficulties at school, even though he did not really like school; he preferred helping his father with the farming. Manuel completed primary and

(continues)

CASE ILLUSTRATIONS   *(continued)*

secondary school in Mexico. Before the alleged incident of incest, he attended several months of school in the U.S. but that was insubstantial. Manuel has no history of drug use. He did acknowledge that shortly before the abuse incident, he started drinking alcohol provided for him by his brothers, who normally drink one or two beers after work.

Although it was difficult for him to talk about it, Manuel did admit he had sexually abused his niece. He talked openly with the examiner about the offense, providing full details and taking full responsibility for his behavior. He expressed regret and remorse for having harmed his niece and his family by his actions. He reported that he did not know he was not supposed to leave the country when he "absconded."

In Deciding How to Respond to This Case, Consider:

- What might help you determine whether a culturally competent evaluation had been performed by the examiner?
- What cultural factors should be taken into account in appropriately assessing Manuel's risk for fleeing the country?
- What cultural elements might an examiner have to consider or be familiar with in order to make an appropriate assessment of the sexual misbehavior?
- How might Manuel's family be used as a resource in treatment?
- What improvements or changes need to be made in Manuel's life to ensure that he will be in the best position possible to make good decisions for himself in the future?
- What you do as a therapist to help ensure that Manuel will stay engaged in treatment?

Response and Recommendation   The prominent cultural factor to be considered in this case is family unity. In talking to Manuel's sister and her husband, they reported that they and all the other siblings were willing to support Manuel through this treatment program. They were well-established in the United States, having bought their own home recently, and the brother-in-law had his own business. Because family unity is particularly strong in Latino culture, and because Manuel has all his brothers and sisters currently living in the U.S., the possibility of Manuel leaving the country is very low. It was recommended that Manuel be released to the custody of his sister and brother-in-law, be placed on probation, and be required to attend outpatient sex-offender treatment. Manuel attended treatment for 30 months and was successfully discharged from probation on his 18th birthday.

ACTION STEPS

It is difficult to pull together all of the information that has been presented in this chapter and the previous ones. It may take some time before all the material presented here comes together for you in your work with Latino clients. It may also be difficult to incorporate all that we have shared with you, all of the time, with all of your Latino clients. Such a comprehensive integration is not expected immediately. The concepts in this text will move between the foreground and background depending on the individual needs of your Latino clients. Therefore, we think it might be helpful to leave you with a list of steps to which you can refer as needed.

- Identify what terminology your client uses to refer to his or her ethnic group membership, both generally and specifically.
- Assess the client's level of ethnic identity; in other words, how salient is the client's ethnic group membership and how relevant is it, from the client's perspective, to the presenting problem?
- Acknowledge the client as an expert on his or her own experience, culturally and otherwise. State what you can bring to the relationship (education and training in psychology, experience, multicultural training, etc.) to complement the client's expertise.
- If an assessment is needed, assure that it is conducted appropriately with regard to language and culture.
- Identify potential resources from the client's ethnic background. Generate these ideas together. What strengths does the client's culture provide for resolving the presenting problem?
- What are the cultural scripts/values that are relevant to understanding the client's presenting problem and in generating a course of treatment?
- Identify potential conflicts between the client's ethnic background and mainstream U.S. culture that may be contributing to the problem or which may be an obstacle in resolving the issue.
- Work together with the client to integrate the client's Latino cultural values with the demands of successfully participating in mainstream U.S. culture.
- Identify any immediate needs that the client may have so that she or he does not leave the first session without some "symptom relief" if needed.
- Explore your own biases about Latino culture that may interfere with effective treatment.
- Is there a need for advocacy or working "out of the box" in some fashion?
- How can you promote personalismo and confianza in the counseling relationship?
- What are the real barriers, such as discrimination, that may be involved in the client's case?

CHAPTER 6

Resource List for Further Reading

ASSESSMENT TOOLS FOR CLINICAL WORK OR RESEARCH

(This is not a comprehensive list; there are other resources, not only in the United States, but available internationally from Spain and other Spanish-Speaking countries)

Acculturation

Acculturation Rating Scale for Mexican Americans—II (ARSMA-II): A revision of the original ARSMA Scale. Cuéllar, I., Arnold, B., & Maldonado, R. (1995). Acculturation Rating Scale for Mexican Americans—II: A revision of the original ARSMA Scale. *Hispanic Journal of Behavioral Sciences, 17,* 275–304.

Acculturation Scale (Mexicans, Cubans, Puerto Ricans and Central Americans). Marín, G., Sabogal, F., Marín, B. V., Otero-Sabogal, R., & Perez-Stable, E. J. (1987). Development of a short acculturation scale for Hispanics. *Hispanic Journal of Behavioral Sciences, 9,* 183–205.

Bidimensional Acculturation Scale for Hispanics (BAS). Marín, G., & Gamba, R. J. (1996). A new measurement of acculturation for Hispanics: The Bidimensional Acculturation Scale for Hispanics (BAS). *Hispanic Journal of Behavioral Sciences, 18,* 297–316.

Psychological Acculturation Scale (PAS). Psychological acculturation: Development of a new measure for Puerto Ricans on the U.S. mainland. Tropp, L. R., Erkut, S., Coll, C. G. (1999). *Educational and Psychological Measurement, 59,* 351–367.

Cultural Scripts

Multiphasic Assessment of Cultural Constructs-Short Form (MACC-SF). Cuéllar, I., Arnold, B., & González, G. (1995). Cognitive referents of acculturation: Assessment of cultural constructs in Mexican Americans. *Journal of Community Psychology, 23,* 339–356.

Familism Scale. Steidel, A. G. L., & Contreras, J. M. (2003). A new familism scale for use with Latino populations. *Hispanic Journal of Behavioral Sciences, 25,* 312–330.

Ethnic Identity

The Ethnic Identity Scale (EIS). Umaña-Taylor, A. J., Yazedjian, A., & Bámaca-Gómez, M. (2004). Developing the Ethnic Identity Scale using Eriksonian and social identity principles. *Identity: An International Journal of Theory and Research, 4,* 9–38.

The Multigroup Ethnic Identity Measure (MEIM). Phinney, J. S. (1992). The Multigroup Ethnic Identity Measure: A new scale for use with diverse groups. *Journal of Adolescent Research, 7,* 156–176.

The Multigroup Ethnic Identity Measure-Revised (MEIM-R). Phinney, J. S., & Ong, A. D. (2007). Conceptualization and Measurement of Ethnic Identity: Current Status and Future Directions. *Journal of Counseling Psychology, 54,* 271–281.

Assessment Resources Available in Spanish
Pearson Assessments/PsychCorp

http://www.pearsonassessments.com/pai/ca/cahome.htm

- *Beck Depression Inventory II*
- *Beck Hopelessness Scale*
- *Beck Anxiety Scale*
- *Beck Scale for Suicide Ideation*
- *Cognitive Linguistic Quick Test* (measure of cognitive strengths and weaknesses)
- *Colombia Mental Maturity Scale*
- *Children's PTSD Inventory*
- *Early Childhood Observation System* (measure of academic progress)
- *Early Reading Diagnostic Assessment, Second Edition*
- *Escala de Inteligencia de Wechsler para Adultos—Tercera Edicion (EIWA-III)*
- *Fonología en Español* (a Spanish phonological intervention guide)
- *Naglierei Nonverbal Ability Test-Individual Administration*
- *NEUROPSI-Attention and Memory*
- *NEUROPSI-Evaluación Neuropsicológica Breve en Español*
- *PrimerPASO* (to identify developmental delays)
- *Reading Level Indicator, Spanish*
- *Test de Vocabulario en Imágenes Peabody* (picture vocabulary test)
- *Wechsler Intelligence Scale for Children, Fourth Edition (WISC-IV Spanish)*

Riverside Publishing (800-323-9540)

http://www.riversidepublishing.com/products/bilingual.html

- *Batería III Woodcock-Muñoz* (comprehensive cognitive and achievement battery)
- *Battelle Developmental Inventory, Second Edition*
- *Bilingual Verbal Ability Test*
- *Logramos* (assessment of academic progress/skills)
- *The Woodcock-Muñoz Language Survey, Revised* (a Spanish/English proficiency assessment battery)

Western Psychological Services (800-648-8857)

http://www.wpspublish.com

- *The Spanish Language Assessment Procedure* (measures ability to understand basic concepts)
- *The Tennessee Self-Concept Scale, Spanish Translation*
- *Piers-Harris Children's Self-Concept Scale, Second Edition*
- *Marital Satisfaction Inventory, Revised, Spanish Administration*
- *Stress Profile*
- *Receptive One-Word Picture Vocabulary Test (Bilingual Record Form)*
- *Expressive One-Word Picture Vocabulary Test (Bilingual Record Form)*
- *Parent–Child Relationship Inventory (Spanish Test Form)*

GENERAL INFORMATION ON LATINOS (POLITICAL ISSUES, STATISTICS, SURVEYS)

Latino USA

This radio journal of news and culture is the only national English-language radio program produced from a Latino perspective. It is a production partnership of KUT Radio and the Center for Mexican American Studies at the University of Texas at Austin. Latino USA was launched in 1993 to provide diverse audiences with multiple perspectives on issues affecting Latinos, foster cross-cultural understanding, enhance relationships among Latino communities, and illuminate the richness of Latino cultural and artistic expression. http://www.latinousa.org/

Mexican American Legal Defense and Education Fund (MALDEF)

Founded in 1968 in San Antonio, Texas, the Mexican American Legal Defense and Educational Fund (MALDEF) is the leading nonprofit Latino litigation, advocacy, and educational outreach institution in the United States. MALDEF's mission is to foster sound public policies, laws, and programs to safeguard the civil rights of the 40 million Latinos living in the United States and to empower the Latino community to fully participate in our society. http://www.maldef.org/

Pew Hispanic Center

Founded in 2001, the Pew Hispanic Center is a nonpartisan research organization supported by the Pew Charitable Trusts. Its mission is to improve understanding of the U.S. Hispanic population and to chronicle Latinos' growing impact on the entire nation. http://pewhispanic.org/

The Tomás Rivera Policy Institute (TRPI)

TRPI was founded in 1985 to conduct objective, policy-relevant research, and disseminate results and their implications to decision-makers on key issues affecting Latino communities. www.trpi.org

TRAINING OPPORTUNITIES AND RESOURCES

CETLALIC (Centro Tlahuica de Lenguas e Intercambio Cultural— The Tlahuica Center for Language and Cultural Exchange)

Founded in 1987 as an alternative school integrating intensive study of Spanish language with experiential cultural learning and analysis of contemporary issues. At CETLALIC, you'll learn Spanish in a friendly atmosphere while expanding your knowledge of the region's cultural, socio-economic, and political realities, making connections between your own country and Mexico/Latin America today. http://www.cetlalic.org.mx/

Del Dicho al Hecho by Profesor Esteban Giménez

An extensive list of dichos (sayings) in Spanish. The English translation or comparable saying is given as well as the significance of the saying.

http://www.belcart.com/belcart_es/del_dicho/indice%20dichos.html

National Latino/a Psychological Association

The National Latina/o Psychological Association (NLPA) is a national organization of mental health professionals and students whose mission is "to generate and advance psychological knowledge and foster its effective application for the benefit of the Hispanic/Latino population." The organization is interested in (a) the mental health needs of individuals who live in the U.S. and have a Latina/o background and (b) addressing the clinical work, research, training and teaching of our members to better serve those individuals.

http://www.nlpa.ws/

MENTAL HEALTH INFORMATION

National Latino Behavioral Health Association (NLBHA)

Established to fill a need for a unified national voice for Latino populations in the behavioral health arena and to bring attention to the great disparities that exist in areas of access, use, practice-based research, and adequately trained personnel. http://www.nlbha.org/

RESOURCES FOR WORKING WITH LATINO CHILDREN

El Corazón de Tejas

The Central Texas Chapter of REFORMA has developed a book list of children's titles with Latino cultural themes. The titles are divided into sections for English, Spanish, and bilingual books and includes bibliographic information to assist in purchasing. Many of the books are available in multiple languages and formats. The list is on the El Corazón de Tejas web site at *http://www.main.org/reforma/Lists/readinglist.html*

HEALTHCARE INFORMATION FOR CLIENTS IN SPANISH

http://www.psiquiatria.com/

A web site with information in Spanish about different mental health disorders.

http://www.ncfh.org/?pid=154

Bilingual Patient Education Materials: general health information created by the National Center for Farm Workers.

http://medlineplus.gov/spanish/

Extensive health topics listed alphabetically with links to Spanish brochures arranged under each topic.

http://www.noah-health.org/

Spanish/English health information site with search engine, browsing access, and links to additional sources.

http://www.ohsu.edu/library/hoodriver/pamphlets/pamphletindex.shtml

OHSU/Hood River Community Health Outreach Project: low literacy pamphlets on dental care, immunization, premature labor, and poison control.

http://www.texmed.org/Template.aspx?id=4388

Texas Medical Association Patient Education Page: this subject list leads to many English and Spanish patient education pamphlets. Even though they are brief, the coverage is very broad.

http://www.niaaa.nih.gov/Publications/PamphletsBrochuresPosters/Spanish/

National Institute on Alcohol Abuse and Alcoholism: pamphlets on alcohol abuse in PDF and HTML formats.

http://www.cdc.gov/spanish/bebe.htm

Center for Disease Control Spanish pamphlets on infant care, adolescent health disease prevention, dental care, and mental health.

http://www.parenting-ed.org/parent-handouts.asp

Parenting Information Handouts: pamphlets in English and Spanish on parenting topics, developed by Arkansas Children's Hospital.

http://www.aacap.org/cs/forFamilies

American Academy of Child and Adolescent Psychiatry: fact sheets on mental health for children and adolescents.

http://www.samhsa.gov/espanol/

Substance Abuse and Mental Health Services Administration: site includes information on children's mental health and intervention skills for parents and teachers.

http://www.nimh.nih.gov

National Institute of Mental Health: pamphlets about mental health in HTML formats.

http://www.womenshealth.gov/espanol/publicaciones/

National Women's Health Information Center: pamphlets and organization sites on alcohol, arthritis, asthma/allergies, cancer, diabetes, diet, drug abuse, mental health, urologic disorders, STDs, and domestic violence.

REFERENCES

Acuña, R. (1972). *Occupied America: The Chicano struggle toward liberation.* San Francisco: Canfield Press.

Alan Guttmacher Institute (2004). U.S. teenage pregnancy statistics: Overall trends, trends by race and ethnicity and state-by-state information. Retrieved December 28, 2005 from www.guttmacher.org/pubs/state_pregnancy_trends.pdf

Alegría, M., Canino, G., Shrout, P. E., Woo, M., Duan, N., Vila, D., ... Meng, X. –L. (2008). Prevalence of mental illness in immigrant and non-immigrant U.S. Latino groups. *American Journal of Psychiatry, 165,* 359–369. doi:10.1176/appi.ajp.2007.07040704

Alicea, M. (1994). The Latino immigration experience: The case of Mexicans, Puertorriqueños, and Cubanos. In N. Kanellos & C. Esteva-Fabregat (Eds.), *Handbook of Hispanic cultures in the United States: Sociology* (pp. 35–56). Houston, TX: Arte Publico Press.

Allen, M. L., Elliott, M. N., Fugligni, A. J., Morales, L. S., Hambarsoomian, K., & Schuster, M. A. (2008). The relationship between Spanish language use and substance use behaviors among Latino youth: A social network approach. *Journal of Adolescent Health, 42,* 372–379. doi:10.1016/j.jadohealth.2008.02.016

Allende, C. A. (2010, Augosto). Ratifica corte: bodas gay válidas en el páis. *El Universal.* Retrieved from http://www.eluniversal.com.mx/notas/700789.html

Altarriba, J., & Bauer, L. (1998). Counseling the Hispanic client: Cuban Americans, Mexican Americans, and Puerto Ricans. *Journal of Counseling and Development, 76,* 389–396.

Amaro, H., Russo, N. F., & Johnson, J. (1987). Family and work predictors of psychological well-being among Hispanic women professionals. *Psychology of Women Quarterly, 11,* 505–521.

American Psychiatric Association (2000). *Diagnostic and statistical manual of mental disorders* (4th ed., Text Rev.) Arlington, VA: Author.

Barnett, T. L. (2004). *Immigration from South America.* Philadelphia: Mason Crest Publishers.

Barrett, B. (1998). Gay and Lesbian activism: A frontier in social advocacy. In *Social action: A mandate for counselors* (pp. 83–98). Alexandria, VA: American Counseling Association.

Beltrán, G. A. (1989). *La población negra de Mexico: estudio etnohistorico* (The Black population of Mexico: An ethnohistorical study). México City: Fondo de Cultura Económica.

Beltrán, I. S. (2005). *The relation of culture to differences in depressive symptoms and coping strategies: Mexican American and European American college students.* Unpublished doctoral dissertation, University of Texas, Austin.

Bennet, H. (2003). *Africans in the colonial Mexico: Absolutism, Christianity, and Afro-Creole consciousness, 1570–1640.* Bloomington, IN: Indiana University Press.

Bryant-Davis, T., & Ocampo, C. (2005). Racist incident-based trauma. *The Counseling Psychologist, 33,* 479–500.

Cardemil, E. V., Kim, S. Pinedo, T. M., Miller, I. W. (2005). Developing a culturally appropriate depression prevention program: The Family Coping Skills Program. *Cultural Diversity & Ethnic Minority Psychology, 11,* 99–112.

Carrillo, C. (1978). Directions for Chicano Psychotherapy. *Spanish Speaking Mental Health Research Center Monograph Series, 7,* 143–156.

Carroll, P. (1991). *Blacks in colonial Veracruz: Race, ethnicity, and regional development.* Austin, TX: University of Texas Press.

Carter, R. T. (1997). Is white a race? Expressions of white racial identity. In M. Fine, L. Weis, L. C. Powell, L. M. Wong (Eds.), *Off White: Readings on Race, Power, and Society* (pp. 198–209). New York: Routledge.

Casas, J. M., & Pytluk, S. D. (1995). Hispanic identity development: Implications for research and practice. In J. G. Ponterotto., J. M. Casas, L. A. Suzuki, & C. M. Alexander (Eds.), *Handbook of multicultural counseling* (pp. 155–180). Thousand Oaks, CA: Sage.

Chase, C. S. (2000). Costa Rican Americans. In Lehman, J. (Ed.), *Gale encyclopedia of multicultural America: Second Edition* (ebook: pp. 429–436). Farmington Hill, Michigan: Gale Group.

Chen, G., LePhuoc, P., Guzmán, M. R., Rude, S., & Dodd, B. (2006). Exploring the complexity of Asian American racial identity. *Cultural Diversity and Ethnic Minority Psychology, 12,* 461–476.

Clark, W. A. V. (2001). *Immigration and Hispanic Middle Class.* Retrieved August 15, 2004 from http://www.cis.org/articles/2001/hispanicmc/toc.html

Cokley, K. (2007). Critical issues in the measurement of ethnic and racial identity: A referendum on the state of the field. *Journal of Counseling Psychology, 54,* 224–234.

Comas-Díaz, L. (2001). Hispanics, Latinos, or Americanos: The evolution of identity. *Cultural Diversity and Ethnic Minority Psychology, 7,* 115–120.

Costantino, G., Malgady, R. G., & Rogler, L. H. (1986). Cuento therapy: A culturally sensitive modality for Puerto Rican children. *Journal of Consulting and Clinical Psychology, 54,* 639–645.

Cross, W. E., Jr. (1995). The psychology of Nigrescence: Revising the Cross model. In J. G. Ponterotto., J. M. Casas, L. A. Suzuki, & C. M. Alexander (Eds.), *Handbook of multicultural counseling* (pp. 93–122). Thousand Oaks, CA: Sage.

Cross, W. E., Jr., & Vandiver, B. J. (2001). Nigrescence theory and measurement: Introducing the Cross Racial Identity Scale (CRIS). In J. G. Ponterotto., J. M. Casas, L. A. Suzuki, & C. M. Alexander (Eds.), *Handbook of multicultural counseling* (2nd ed., pp. 371–393). Thousand Oaks, CA: Sage.

Cuéllar, I., Arnold, B., & González, G. (1995). Cognitive referents of acculturation: Assessment of cultural constructs in Mexican Americans. *Journal of Community Psychology, 23,* 339–356.

Cuéllar, I., Arnold, B., & Maldonado, R. (1995). Acculturation Rating Scale for Mexican Americans—II: A revision of the original ARSMA Scale. *Hispanic Journal of Behavioral Sciences, 17,* 275–304.

Davis, D. J. (Ed.) (1995). *Slavery and beyond: The African impact on Latin American and the Caribbean.* Wilmington, DE: Scholarly Resources Inc.

De Genova, N., & Ramos-Zayas, A. Y. (2003). *Latino crossings: Mexicans, Puerto Ricans, and the politics of race and citizenship.* New York: Routledge.

Diaz, R. M., Ayala, G., Bein, D. E., Henne, J., & Marin, B. V. (2001). The impact of homophobia, poverty, and racism on the mental health of gay and bisexual Latino men: Findings from three U.S. cities. *American Journal of Public Health, 91,* 927–932.

Dingfelder, S. F. (January, 2005). Closing the gap for Latino patients. *Monitor on Psychology.* Washington, DC: American Psychological Association.

Duany, J. (2002). *Puerto Rican nation on the move: Identities on the island and in the United States.* Chapel Hill, NC: University of North Carolina Press.

Durand, J. (2004). *From traitors to heroes: 100 years of Mexican migration policies.* Washington D.C.: Migration Policy Institute.

Espinosa, G., Elizondo, V., and Miranda, J. (2003). *Hispanic Churches in American Public Life: Summary of Findings.* Notre Dame, IN: Institute for Latino Studies. Retrieved December 28, 2005 from http://www.nd.edu/~latino/research/pubs/HispChurchesEnglishWEB.pdf

Falicov, C. J. (1998). *Latino families in therapy.* New York: Guilford Press.

Finch, B. K., Kolody, B., & Vega, W. A. (2000). Perceived discrimination and depression among Mexican-origin adults in California. *Journal of Health & Social Behavior, 41,* 295–313.

Fitzpatrick, J. P. (1987). *Puerto Rican Americans: The meaning of migration to the mainland.* Englewood Cliffs, New Jersey: Prentice-Hall, Inc.

Flores, J. (1993). *Divided borders: Essays on Puerto Rican identity.* Houston: Arte Público Press.

Fraga, E. D., Atkinson, D. R., & Wampold, B. E. (2004). Ethnic group preferences for multicultural counseling competencies. *Cultural Diversity & Ethnic Minority Psychology, 10,* 53–65.

Fukuyama, M. A., & Sevig, T. D. (2002). Spirituality in counseling across cultures. In *Counseling Across Cultures* (5th ed., pp. 273–295). Thousand Oaks, CA: Sage.

Galan, H. (Producer/Director). (2000). *The forgotten Americans.* [Motion Picture]. San Marcos, TX: Southwest Texas State University.

García, M. C. (1996). *Havana USA.* Berkley, University of California Press.

García y Griego, M. (1996). The importation of Mexican contract laborers to the United States, 1942–1964. In Gutiérrez, D. G. (Ed.), *Between two worlds: Mexican immigrants in the United States.* Wilmington, Delaware: SR Book.

Gil, R. M., and Vazquez, C. I. (1996). *The Maria Paradox: How Latinas can merge old world traditions with new world self-esteem.* New York: Berkley Publishing Group.

Gonzales, M. G. (2000). *Mexicanos: A history of Mexican Americans in the United States.* Bloomington, Indiana: Indiana University Press.

Gonzales, M. G., & Gonzales, C. M. (2000). *En aquel entonces: Readings in Mexican American history.* Bloomington, Indiana: Indiana University Press.

Gonzales, R. (1967). *I am Joaquin: An epic poem.* New York: Bantam Books.

Gonzalez, D. (1992, November). What's the problem with 'Hispanic'? Just ask a 'Latino.' *The New York Times,* Section 4, p. 6.

Gonzalez, J. (2000). *Harvest of Empire: A history of Latinos in America.* New York: Penguin Books.

Granados, C. (2000, December). *Hispanic vs. Latino.* Hispanic, 39–42.

Green, D. (2000). Puerto Rican Americans. In Lehman, J. (Ed.), *Gale Encyclopedia of Multicultural America: Second Edition* (ebook: pp. 1489–1503). Farmington Hill, Michigan: Gale Group.

Grenier, G. J., & Pérez, L. (2003). *The Legacy of Exile: Cubans in the United States.* Boston, Massachusetts: Allyn & Bacon.

Grieco, E. (2003). *The Foreign Born from Mexico in the United States.* Washington D.C.: Migration Policy Institute.

Grieco, E. (2004). *The Foreign Born from the Dominican Republic in the United States*. Washington D.C.: Migration Policy Institute.

Guarnero, P. A., & Flaskerud, J. H. (2008). Latino gay men and depression. *Issues in Mental Health Nursing, 29*, 667–670.

Gutiérrez, D. G. (1996). *Between Two Worlds: Mexican Immigrants in the United States*. Wilmington, Delaware: SR Book.

Guzmán, B. (2001). *The Hispanic population. Census 2000 brief*. C2KBR/01-3. Washington, DC: U.S. Census Bureau.

Guzmán, M. R., Keith, T. Z., & Rico, V. *Ethnic identity and ethnic self-identification in Mexican origin adolescents*. Unpublished manuscript.

Hambleton, R. K., & Patsula, L. (1999). Increasing the validity of adapted tests: Myths to be avoided and guidelines for improving test adaptation practices. *Journal of Applied Testing Technology, 1*, 1–30.

Hagan, J., & Rodriguez, N. (1996). "Central Americans in the United States." *Center for Immigration Research: Working Paper Series*. Houston: University of Houston, College of Social Sciences, Center for Immigration Research.

Hayes-Bautista, D. E., & Chapa, J. (1987). Latino terminology: Conceptual bases for standardized terminology. *American Journal of Public Health, 77*, 61–68.

Helms, J. E. (1995). An update of Helm's white and people of color racial identity models. In J. G. Ponterotto, J. M. Casas, L. A. Suzuki, & C. M. Alexander (Eds.), *Handbook of Multicultural Counseling* (pp. 181–198). Thousand Oaks, CA: Sage.

Hendricks, G. (1974). *The Dominican Diaspora: From the Dominican Republic to New York City—villagers in transition*. New York: Teacher College Press.

Hernandez, R. (2004). *Immigration from Central America*. Philadelphia: Mason Crest Publishers.

Hogg Foundation for Mental Health (2010a). *Integrated Health Care: Connecting Body and Mind*. Retrieved from http://www.hogg.utexas.edu/initiatives/integrated_health_care.html

Hogg Foundation for Mental Health (2010b). *2006 IHC Questions and Answers: Collaborative Care Model*. Retrieved from http://www.hogg.utexas.edu/initiatives/collaborative_care_qa.html

Hong, M. (2000). Guatemalan Americans. In Lehman, J. (Ed.), *Gale encyclopedia of Multicultural America: Second Edition* (ebook: pp. 764–782). Farmington Hill, Michigan: Gale Group.

Itzigsohn, J., Giorguli, S., & Vazquez, O. (2005). Immigrant incorporation and racial identity: Racial self-identification among Dominican immigrants, *Ethnic and Racial Studies, 28*, 50–78.

Jenkins, J. H. (1988). Conceptions of schizophrenia as a problem of nerves: A cross-cultural comparison of Mexican Americans and Anglo Americans. *Social Science and Medicine, 26*, 1233–1243.

Johnston, F. (1981). *The Wonder of Guadalupe: The origin and cult of the miraculous image of the Blessed Virgin in Mexico*. Rockford, IL: Tan Books and Publishers.

Kanel, K. (2002). Mental health needs of Spanish-speaking Latinos in southern California. *The Hispanic Journal of Behavioral Sciences, 24*, 74–91.

Keigwin, A. J. (2005). *Assembly Passes Bill to End the Use of Children as Interpreters in Medical Situations*. News from the 12th Assembly District. Retrieved on January 6, 2006 from http://democrats.assembly.ca.gov/members/a12/press/p122005052.htm

Kerwin, C., & Ponterotto, J. G. (1995). Biracial identity development: Theory and research. In J. G. Ponterotto, J. M. Casas, L. A. Suzuki, & C. M. Alexander (Eds.), *Handbook of Multicultural Counseling* (pp. 199–217). Thousand Oaks, CA: Sage.

Kester E. S., & Peña E. (2002). Language ability assessment of Spanish–English bilinguals: Future Direction. Retrieved February, 6, 2006 from *Practical Assessment, Research and Evaluation, 8*, http://pareonline.net/Home.htm.

Kochhar, R. (2004). *Pew Hispanic Center Report: The Wealth of Hispanic Households: 1996–2002*. Retrieved from http://pewhispanic.org/files/reports/34.pdf

Korrol, V. (1994). In their own right: A history of Puerto Ricans in the U.S.A. In N. Kanellos & C. Esteva-Fabregat (Eds.), *Handbook of Hispanic Cultures in the United States: History* (pp. 281–301). Houston, TX: Arte Público Press.

Kristo, E. (2009, March). A portrait of integrated health care in El Paso. Hogg Foundation for Mental Health. Retrieved from http://www.hogg.utexas.edu/detail/61/Project_Vida.html

LaFromboise, T., Coleman, H. L. K., & Gerton, J. (1993). Psychological impact of biculturalism: Evidence and theory. *Psychological Bulletin, 114*, 395–412.

Lencheck, S. (1997). La Malinche—harlot or heroine? Mexico History, December 1997: "El Ojo del Lago," Guadalajara-Lakeside Volume 14, Number 4. Retrieved from www.mexconnect.com/articles/224-la-malinche-harlot-or-heroine

Lopez-Baez, S. I. (1997). Counseling interventions with Latinas. In *Multicultural issues in counseling, new approaches to diversity*, 2nd edition, C. C. Lee. Alexandria, VA: American Counseling Association.

Los Reyes Magos (The Three Kings). (2005, December 18). *El Boricua*. Retrieved on December 29, 2005 from http://www.elboricua.com/losreyes.html

MALDEF (2010). *Court Blocks Major Provisions of Arizona's Anti-Immigrant Law*. Retrieved from http://maldef.org/news/releases/court_blocks_major_07282010/

Mainous, A. G., III, Diaz, V. A., & Geesey, M. E. (2008). Acculturation and healthy lifestyle among Latinos with diabetes. *Annals of Family Medicine, 6*, 131–137. doi:10.1370/afm.814

Marrero, P. (2009). What health care reform means for Latinos. New American Media. Retrieved From http://news.newamericamedia.org/news/view_article.html?article_id=569cecc20e31e100-ce297b888c00be8e

Martínez, O. J. (Ed.). (1996). *U.S.–Mexico borderlands: Historical and contemporary perspectives*. Wilmington, DE: Scholarly Resources Inc.

McKissack, F., & McKissack P. (1996). *Rebels against slavery: American slave revolts*. New York: Scholastic.

McWilliams, C. (1968). *North from Mexico*. New York: Greenwood Press.

Meier, M., & Rivera, F. (1972) *The Chicanos: A History of Mexican Americans*. New York: Hill and Wang.

Melville, M. B. (1994). "Hispanics" ethnicity, race and class. In Kanellos, N., & Esteva-Fabregat, C. (Eds.), *Handbook of Hispanic Cultures in the United States: Sociology* (pp. 84–104). Houston, TX: Arte Publico Press.

Miranda, J., Azocar, F., Organista, K. C., Dwyer, E., & Areane, P. (2003). Treatment of depression among impoverished primary care patients from ethnic minority groups. *Psychiatric Services, 54,* 219–225.

Miranda, J., Azocar, F., Organista, K. C., Muñoz, R. F., & Lieberman, A. (1996). Recruiting and retaining low-income Latinos in psychotherapy research. *Journal of Consulting and Clinical Psychology, 64,* 868–874.

Miranda, J., Schoenbaum, M., Sherbourne, C., Duan, N., & Wells, K. (2004). Effects of primary care depression treatment on minority patients' clinical status and employment. *Archives of General Psychiatry, 61, 827–834.*

Mirandé, A. (1985). *The Chicano experience: An alternative perspective.* Notre Dame, Indiana: University of Notre Dame Press.

National Campaign to Prevent Teen Pregnancy (2005, November). *Teen Sexual Activity, Pregnancy and Childbearing among Latinos in the United States.* Washington, DC: The National Campaign to Prevent Teen Pregnancy. Retrieved December 28, 2005 from http:// www.teenpregnancy.org/ resources/reading/pdf/latinofs.pdf

Neff, A. J., & Hoppe, S. K. (1993). Race/ethnicity, acculturation and psychological distress: Fatalism and religiosity as cultural resources. *Journal of Community Psychology, 21,* 3–20.

Niemann, Y. F. (2001). Stereotypes about Chicanas and Chicanos: Implications for counseling. *The Counseling Psychologist, 29,* 55–90.

Novas, H. (1998). *Everything you need to know about Latino History.* New York: Plume.

Ochoa, G. (2001). *Atlas of Hispanic American history.* New York: Checkmark Books.

Office of Immigration Statistics (2010). *2009 Yearbook of Immigration Statistics.* Retrieved from http://www. dhs.gov/xlibrary/assets/statistics/ yearbook/2009/ois_yb_2009.pdf

Ogbu, J. U. (1987). Variability in minority school performance: A problem in search of an explanation. *Anthropology & Education Quarterly, 18,* 312–334.

Opler, L. A., Ramirez, P. M., Dominguez, L., Fox, M. S., & Johnson, P. B. (2004). Rethinking medication prescribing practices in an inner-city Hispanic mental health clinic. *Journal of Psychiatric Practice, 10,* 134–140.

Pecquet, J. (2010). White House highlights healthcare reform benefits for Latinos. Healthwatch, The Hill's Healthcare Blog, The Hill. Retrieved from http://thehill.com/ blogs/healthwatch/health-reform-implementation/117621-white-house–highlights-health-reform-para-latinos

Pessar, P. R. (1995). *A Visa for a Dream: Dominicans in the United States.* Boston: Allyn & Bacon.

Pessar, P. R., & Graham, P. R. (2001). Dominicans: Transnational identities and local politics. In Foner, N. (ed.), *New Immigrants to New York.* New York: Colombia University Press.

Pew Hispanic Center (2009). Fact Sheet. *Hispanics of Dominican Origin in the United States, 2007.* Retrieved from http://pewhispanic. org/files/factsheets/52.pdf

Pew Hispanic Center (2010). *Statistical Portrait of Hispanics in the United States.* Retrieved from http:// pewhispanic.org/reports/report. php?ReportID=120

Pew Hispanic Center & Kaiser Family Foundation (2002, December). *2002 National survey of Latinos.* Retrieved from http://www. pewhispanic.org/index.jsp

Phinney, J. S. (1990). Ethnic identity in adolescents and adults: Review of research. *Psychological Bulletin, 108,* 499–514.

Phinney, J. S. (1992). The Multigroup Ethnic Identity Measure: A new scale for use with diverse groups. *Journal of Adolescent Research, 7,* 156–176.

Phinney, J. S. (1996). Understanding ethnic diversity: The role of ethnic identity. *American Behavioral Scientist, 40,* 143–152.

Phinney, J. S., & Ong, A. D. (2007). Conceptualization and Measurement of Ethnic Identity: Current Status and Future Directions.

Journal of Counseling Psychology, 54, 271–281.

Pole, N., Best, S. R., Metzler, T., & Marmar, C. R. (2005). Why are Hispanics at greater risk for PTSD? *Cultural Diversity and Ethnic Minority Psychology, 11,* 144–161.

Ponterotto, J. (1987). Counseling Mexican Americans: A Multimodal Approach. *Journal of Counseling and Development, 65,* 308–312.

Poyo, G., & Diaz-Miranda, M. (1994). Cubans in the United States. In N. Kanellos & C. Esteva-Fabregat (Eds.), *Handbook of Hispanic Cultures in the United States: History* (pp. 303–320). Houston, TX: Arte Público Press.

Ramirez, R. R., & de la Cruz, G. P. (2002). The Hispanic population in the United States. *Current Population Reports,* P20–545, Washington, DC: U.S. Census Bureau.

Ramos, J. (2004). *The Latino Wave.* New York: HarperCollins Publishers Inc.

Raul Castro named Cuban president. (2008, February). BBC News. Retrieved from http://news.bbc.co. uk/2/hi/americas/7261204.stm

Reid, F. (Producer/Director/Writer), & Wood, S. (Writer). (1995). *Skin deep* [Motion Picture]. Berkeley, CA: Iris Films.

Ricourt, M. (2002). *Dominicans in New York: Power from the margin.* London: Routledge.

Rodriguez, J. (2000). Argentinean Americans. In Lehman, J. (Ed.), *Gale encyclopedia of Multicultural America: Second Edition* (ebook: pp. 123–132). Farmington Hill, Michigan: Gale Group.

Rodriguez, R. (1982). *Hunger of Memory: The education of Richard Rodriguez.* New York: Bantam Books. 1982.

Rodriguez, C. E., & Korrol, V. S. (Eds.). (1996). *Historical perspectives on Puerto Rican survival in the U.S.* Princeton, NJ: Markus Wiener Publishers.

Rodriguez, R. R., & Walls, N. E. (2000). Culturally educated questioning: Toward a skills-based approach in multicultural counselor training. *Applied & Preventive Psychology, 9,* 89–99.

Rosenthal Gelman, C. (2004). Toward a better understanding of the use of psychodynamically-informed treatment with Latinos: Findings from clinician experience. *Clinical Social Work, 32,* 61–77.

Rotter, J. B. (1990). Internal versus external control of reinforcement: A case history of a variable. *American Psychologist, 45,* 489–493.

Sánchez, G. J. (1993). *Becoming Mexican American: ethnicity, culture, and identity in Chicano Los Angeles.* New York: Oxford University Press.

Santiago, E. (1993). *When I was Puerto Rican.* New York: Vintage Books.

Santiago-Rivera, A. L. (1995). Developing a culturally sensitive treatment modality for bilingual Spanish-speaking clients: Incorporating culture and language in therapy. *Journal of Counseling and Development, 74,* 12–17.

Santiago-Rivera, A. L. & Altarriba, J. (2002). The role of language in therapy with the Spanish-English bilingual client. *Professional Psychology: Research and Practice, 33,* 30–38.

Santiago-Rivera, A. L., Arredondo, P., & Gallardo-Cooper, M. (2002). *Counseling Latinos and La Familia: A practical guide.* Thousand Oaks, CA: Sage.

Schaefer, R. T. (2002). *Racial and Ethnic Groups: Census 2000 update.* Upper Saddle River, New Jersey: Prentice-Hall.

Schwartz, S. J., Unger, J. B., Zamboanga, B. L., Szapocznik, J. (2010). Rethinking the concept of acculturation: Implications for theory and research. *American Psychologist, 65,* 237–251.

Smagula, S. (2000). Nicaraguan Americans. In Lehman, J. (Ed.), *Gale Encyclopedia of Multicultural America: Second Edition* (ebook: pp. 1295–1310). Farmington Hill, Michigan: Gale Group.

Southern Poverty Law Center (2010). Anti-immigrant hate crimes. *Intelligence Report.* Retrieved from http://www.splcenter.org/ intelligence-report/-year-hate/ anti-immigrant-hate-crimes

Suarez-Orozco, C., & Suarez-Orozco, M. M. (1995). *Transformations: Immigration, family life, and achievement motivation among Latino adolescents.* Stanford, CA: Stanford University Press.

Sue, D. W., Arredondo, P., & McDavis, R. J. (1992). Multicultural competencies/standards: A pressing need. *Journal of Counseling and Development, 70,* 477–486.

Sue, D. W., Capodilupo, C. M., Torino, G. C., Bucceri, J. M., Holder, A. M. B., Nadal, K. L., & Esquilin, M. (2007). Racial microaggressions in everyday life. *American Psychologist, 62,* 271–286.

Sue, D. W., & Sue, S. (2003). *Counseling the Culturally Diverse, Theory and Practice* (4th ed.) New York: John Wiley & Sons.

Suro, R. (2002). *Counting the "Other Hispanics": How many Colombians, Dominicans, Ecuadorians, Guatemalans, and Salvadorans are there in the United States?* Washington D.C.: Pew Hispanic Center.

Takeuchi, D. T., Sue, S., & Yeh, M. (1995). Return rates and outcomes from ethnicity-specific mental health programs in Los Angeles. *American Journal of Public Health, 85,* 638–643.

Thomas, P. (1967). *Down these Mean Streets.* New York: Random House.

Umaña-Taylor, A. J., Yazedjian, A., & Bámaca-Gómez, M. (2004). Developing the Ethnic Identity Scale using Eriksonian and social identity principles. *Identity: An International Journal of Theory and Research, 4,* 9–38.

Unger, J. B., Reynolds, K., Shakib, S., Spruijt-Metz, D., Sun, P., & Johnson, C. A. (2004). Acculturation, physical activity and fast-food consumption among Asian-Americans and Hispanic adolescents. *Journal of Community Health, 29,* 467–481. doi:10.1007/ s10900-004-3395-3.

U.S. Census Bureau (2010a, July). Facts for Features. *Hispanic Heritage Month 2010: Sept. 15 — Oct. 15.* Retrieved from http://www.census. gov/newsroom/releases/archives/ facts_for_features_special_ editions/cb10-ff17.html

U.S. Census Bureau (2010b). *The 2010 Statistical Abstract. Table 224. Educational Attainment by Race and Hispanic Origin: 1970 to 2008.* Retrieved from http://www.census. gov/compendia/statab/2010/tables/ 10s0224.pdf

U.S. Census Bureau (2010c). *The 2010 Statistical Abstract. Table 227. Mean Earnings by Highest Degree Earned: 2007.* Retrieved from http://www. census.gov/compendia/statab/ 2010/tables/10s0227.pdf

U.S. Department of Commerce, Bureau of the Census (2000). *Short Form Questionnaire: Informational Short Form Questionnaire* [PDF].

Retrieved from http://www.census. gov/dmd/www/2000quest.html

U.S. Department of Health and Human Services (2001). *Mental Health: Culture, Race, and Ethnicity—A supplement to mental health: A report of the surgeon general.* Rockville, MD: U.S. Department of Health and Human Services, Substance Abuse and Mental Health Services Administration, Center for Mental Health Services. Retrieved from http://www.mentalhealth. samhsa.gov/cre/toc.asp

U.S. Department of Labor, Bureau of Labor Statistics (2003). Unemployment in 2002 by Race, Hispanic Ethnicity, and Sex. Retrieved from http://www.bls.gov/opub/ted/2003/ dec/wk5/art01.htm

U.S. Department of Labor, Bureau of Labor Statistics (2010a). *Economic News Release. Table A-2. Employment status of the civilian population by race, sex and age.* Retrieved from http://www.bls.gov/news.release/ empsit.t02.htm

U.S. Department of Labor, Bureau of Labor Statistics (2010b). *Economic News Release. Table A-3. Employment Status of the Hispanic or Latino Population by Sex and Age.* Retrieved from http://www.bls. gov/news.release/empsit.t03.htm

Valdes, M. (1983). Psychotherapy with Hispanics. *Psychotherapy in Private Practice, 1,* 55–62.

Vandiver, B. J., Fhagen-Smith, P. E., Cokley, K., Cross, W. E., Jr., & Worrell, F. C. (2001) Cross' nigrescence model: From theory to scale to theory. *Journal of Multicultural Counseling and Development, 29,* 174–200.

Vasconcelos, J. (1979). *The Cosmic Race/La raza cosmica.* Los Angles: California State University.

Vega, W. A., & Lopez, S. R. (2001). Priority issues in Latino mental health services research. *Mental Health Services Research, 3,* 189–199.

Villaseñor, V. (2004). *Burro Genius.* New York: HarperCollins Publishers Inc.

Wade, M. (1995). *Cabeza de Vaca: Conquistador who cared.* Houston, TX: Colophon House.

Weaver, T. (1994). The culture of Latinos in the United States. In J. N. Kanellos & C. Esteva-Fabregat (Eds.), *Handbook of Hispanic Cultures in the United States: Sociology* (pp. 15–38). Houston, TX: Arte Publico Press.

Wikipedia (2010). Patient Protection and Affordable Care Act. Retrieved from http://en.wikipedia.org/wiki/Patient_Protection_and_Affordable_Care_Act

Williams, D. R., Neighbors, H. W., & Jackson, J. S. (2003). Racial/ethnic discrimination and health: Findings from community studies. *American Journal of Public Health*, 93, 200–208.

Williams, D. R., & Willaims-Morris, R. (2000). Racism and mental health: The African American experience. *Ethnicity & Health*, 5, 1355–7858.

Zúñiga, M. E. (1992). *Dichos* as metaphorical tools for resistant Latino clients. *Psychotherapy*, 28, 480–483.

INDEX

Note: italicized page numbers refer to tables.